# FOODS WITHOUT FADS

*By the Same Author:* BASIC NUTRITION

# Foods Without Fads

## A COMMON SENSE GUIDE
## TO NUTRITION

By E. W. McHenry, Ph.D.

PROFESSOR OF NUTRITION,
SCHOOL OF HYGIENE,
UNIVERSITY OF TORONTO

J. B. LIPPINCOTT COMPANY

PHILADELPHIA / NEW YORK

# Contents

# Contents

# *Preface*

This book is intended to supply reliable information about nutrition and about food choice. In the past 50 years a large amount of scientific information has become available. Much of this has been validated by repeated research. Some more recent reports concern research in progress and cannot yet be accepted as valid. One of the major problems in modern life is to provide scientific information in a clear form which can be understood by persons without scientific training. While misinformation is available in various fields, nutrition is particularly confused by pseudo experts and by some popular writers. Reports of current research are frequently presented as finished business; unfortunately, this is not always right. The author has endeavored to present simply and clearly statements about nutrition which are supported by considerable evidence.

I have been assisted greatly by my wife, who is the practising nutritionist in our home, by my secretary, Miss Jewel Chadwell, and by the staff of the publishers.

E. W. McHenry

# CHAPTER 1

# *Why Eat Food? To Satisfy Hunger or to Conform to Custom?*

Hunger is the primary reason for eating food, but on many occasions people eat when they are not hungry. Social obligations may cause food to be consumed to avoid giving offense even if hunger is absent. Primitive man may have eaten only when he was hungry but civilization has caused many changes. Eating meals in family, or larger, groups may have developed early in human history and eating took on the aspect of a social occasion. On special feast days customs evolved regarding the use of special foods and of elaborate meals. The times for meals changed with the growth of industry and of large cities. Artificial light made possible mealtimes which were impossible when daylight was the only illumination. Particular foods became associated with individual meals. The types of foods eaten often vary from one race to another and from one area to another, and people become accustomed to certain foods in meals and to eating because it is the custom. Dogs, living with humans, acquire taste for human foods and eat when the family is eating.

Despite custom, hunger is the urge to eat and hunger is controlled by a mechanism which functions beautifully in most people and too well in some people. It used to be thought that hunger resulted from emptiness of the stomach. After the development of insulin for the treatment of diabetes, it was observed that, when the amount of sugar in the blood was decreased by administering insulin, hunger developed. Hence, it was concluded that the concentration of sugar in the blood controlled the production of the sensation we call hunger. If the blood sugar is low, hunger develops. If the blood sugar is raised, hunger disappears.

There is no clear-cut explanation of hunger generally accepted by scientists. Several explanations are in vogue at present and these are more complicated than the previous simple ones about the emptiness of the stomach or the concentration of sugar in the blood. Nevertheless, the simple explanations still have practical importance. If sweet food is eaten, the blood sugar is increased and hunger is lessened. This can be seen very clearly if children are given sweet food shortly before a meal; they have little hunger for the meal. Many people like a sweet dessert because it gives them a satisfied feeling that the meal has been sufficient. Emptiness of the stomach is of practical importance, also. Hunger can be lessened by filling the stomach even with material which has very little food value. People who are interested in losing weight are urged to eat bulky, nonfattening foods like some of the vegetables and fruits; these fill the stomach without giving high energy value.

The sensation called hunger is produced in part, at least, by wave-like contractions of the stomach wall. The "pangs of hunger" are felt as a consequence of these contractions. It is now generally assumed that the contractions do not happen only because the stomach is empty; an empty stomach doesn't contract if the nerves leading to the stomach are cut. The stomach contracts as a result of a message carried to it by the nerves. The message originates in a portion of the central nervous system near the brain but actually not part of the brain. This portion is called by an unusual name, hypothalamus, which means under the back of the brain. The next point is, what causes the hypothalamus to send the message to produce hunger? A likely explanation brings in the blood sugar. If sugar is available to the hypothalamus from the blood, the sensation of hunger is not produced. In the period after a meal is eaten, the amount of sugar is increased in the blood, sugar is available to the hypothalamus and it does not send a hunger message. When available sugar has been withdrawn from the blood to feed the various parts of the body, sugar is no longer supplied to the hypothalamus and it sends a message to the stomach, which is empty by that time. Contractions of the stomach wall begin and we feel the sensation of hunger.

This mechanism, which causes us to feel hungry and which impels us to eat, functions, of course, in the reverse direction, also, in most people at the end of a meal. After food has been eaten, blood sugar is increased and hunger is replaced by a feeling of satisfaction. The mechanism can, however, be disturbed and altered by several influences. Smoking tends to lessen hunger and heavy smokers may not eat as much as nonsmokers. Alcohol, in moderation, stimulates hunger and increases the intake of food. A cocktail or a glass of sherry before dinner can cause people to gain weight because of the extra food eaten. Although the alcohol itself is a source of calories, its contribution is usually less than that of the additional food. Unpleasant sights or smells can depress hunger while pleasant smells (like that of freshly baked bread) can stimulate hunger and encourage eating.

Because the mechanism stops the production of the hunger sensation, as well as starting the sensation, the body has a built-in arrangement for keeping us from eating more than we need. However, the stopping of hunger may not work too well in some people. It is said that this is a reason why some people become overweight. They have a control mechanism which is abnormal and they eat more than is needed. It is known that damage produced intentionally to the hypothalamus in experimental animals can so alter the hunger control that the animals eat extraordinary amounts of food and become obese. While a similar situation may occur in humans, there is another aspect of considerable practical importance. Custom, or habit, can influence the hunger control. Social custom can cause us to eat when we are not hungry. We can accustom ourselves to eating enough food to make us feel "comfortable," or distended. If this is done meal after meal for some time we develop a habit of eating to produce distention, and satisfaction over a meal is not felt without distention. This habit of heavy eating can develop in childhood and become so firmly fixed that it is one of the very real problems in reducing weight. People will frequently blame overweight on heredity; actually, the likely explanation is that children do learn from their parents. If the parents are heavy eaters, the children tend to become heavy eaters too. Once the habit of overeating is firmly entrenched it is very difficult to break. Obviously, it is better not to let the habit develop.

While we have some understanding of the mechanism which produces the hunger that causes eating and which can terminate the intake of food (if the mechanism is not influenced by one or more of several factors), hunger control is of much less importance in some parts of the world than in others. Those of us who live in "have" countries may never experience really urgent hunger sensations. We can have breakfast every morning (if we get up in time), we can have substantial lunches and dinners without much concern. How different it is with people in other countries where food is scarce. There the sensation of hunger is urgent and the means of satisfying it very meager. If some of us knew the urgency of real hunger, we might feel quite differently about whether we should bother to have breakfast. Many of us eat breakfast, not because we are hungry, but because it is the custom. We may not be consciously aware of the actual need for breakfast. Custom or habit may decide how much will be eaten and the kinds of foods which will be used.

# CHAPTER 2

# Our Choice of Food: Food Habits

Whether we eat because we are hungry or because of custom, our selection of food depends largely on habits which have been developing since childhood. That doesn't mean that everyone has the same food habits. Nor does it mean that habits cannot be changed. Alterations can take place. Generally speaking, our habits regarding food use can become frightfully rigid as we grow older.

Have you ever thought about your food habits? It is interesting, and useful, to consider our own habits and the influences which formed them. If you have children in the household it is your duty to think about the habits which the children are developing and about your influence on these habits. The habits are likely to last for years and may have a definite bearing on health.

There is certainly a tendency for habits of food use to be passed on from parents to children. This is evident in

14

several ways. The selection of food used in a family is likely to depend on the habits of the dominant person in the family. Mother may do the shopping and the cooking but she is unlikely to buy and prepare food to which father strenuously objects. Of course, it can be mother who makes the decision. Can we expect an eight-year-old boy to drink milk if father states flatly that milk is food for sissies? Or, that he doesn't like cauliflower, has never eaten it, and look what a big man he is? Father's habits of food use may have come from his father. However, family food use is influenced by a number of factors in addition to the likes and dislikes or the established habits of the parents.

Race is commonly thought to have a strong effect on food use. Sometimes that is true but there can be confusion between race and another factor, availability. People who live in southern China, Japan, and other areas in the Far East, are regarded as rice-eaters. Do they eat rice because of race or because rice can be grown in the area in which they live while other cereals cannot be grown? Sometimes particular foods become associated with certain races because of custom and not because of availability. We think of sauerkraut as a German food and spaghetti as Italian.

Religious precepts have a strong influence on the use of food. The eating of meat may be forbidden on certain days or it may not be permitted at any time. Some kinds of meat may be allowed and other kinds not permitted. A sincere member of a religious faith will, of course, be governed in his use of food by the principles of his religion.

Improvements in agriculture, in food preservation, in transportation, and in food processing have made possible many changes in food use. When I was a boy, I saw oranges only at Christmas, when they were a special treat. Now I expect to have an orange or a grapefruit every morning; I never saw a grapefruit when I was a youngster. The growing of oranges and grapefruit has been improved greatly and refrigerated transport makes possible the shipment of fruit over long distances. Fifty years ago milk was distributed in cities in cans from which a quart or so was measured out at the house door. The convenience of bottles or paper containers was unknown and practically no attention was given to the safety or quality of milk. Skim milk can now be processed into a stable powder with excellent storage characteristics and the powder can be shipped into areas where fresh milk is scarce or unavailable. The improvements in canning processes make possible the eating of numerous varieties of fruits and vegetables out-of-season. Frozen foods and even frozen prepared meals are markedly altering food habits. Those of us of middle age or older can look back on many changes in food use.

Our choice of food is influenced by advertising to a greater extent than is sometimes realized. One of the problems in the advertising of foods is the reliability of claims made for the advertised food. Government regulations and the enforcement of those regulations operate primarily for the protection of the consumer but, in the long run, they are in the interest of the manufacturer. False claims may boomerang. Control of advertising claims for foods (and drugs) deserves strong support from all of us. Even the households of food producers buy foods and should be concerned about the real values of different foods.

Notions and folklore information about foods have

had considerable influence on food selection. There was a period of some years in North America during which tomatoes were considered to be poisonous and they were grown in gardens for decoration. The brave souls who tried eating tomatoes must have had a rough time with their neighbors. Then, for some time, some people thought tomatoes were a fruit to be eaten for dessert. Many other false notions about foods will be mentioned later. All of these notions tend to limit food use. Sometimes special virtues are attached to foods. It should be noted that some of these claims are made by financially interested people. People are urged to eat sunflower or millet seeds or molasses not only to preserve health but to cure certain diseases. These claims may keep people from having decent meals but, more seriously, they may keep people from obtaining proper medical attention— this can lead to a worsening of the disease. The hucksters who promote special foods with therapeutic claims have a belief in common with the late P. T. Barnum, that a fool is born every minute.

Food fads have been said to be a serious threat to health. In most cases that is doubtful for several reasons. Fads don't usually last long enough these days to cause much harm except in people who seem to be addicted to following fads and who shift from one to another to keep up with progress. Fortunately, also, dietary fads are taken up by comparatively few people in any community, usually by "educated" people. Perhaps the main harm done by following a fad diet is that people are prevented from eating good meals. The worst of it is that the rest of the household may be involved if one parent is a fad addict. I can remember being praised by several men because I said at a public meeting, when the fad for molasses-yoghurt-wheat germ was at its height, that claims made for that combination were rubbish. The poor fellows were being confronted with these foods because their wives went in for diet fads.

Food prices and the amount of money which families have for the purchase of food can change food selection and, sometimes, long-standing habits. If a particular food becomes expensive as a result of scarcity, consumption is likely to decrease. A severe frost in Florida may cause a substantial increase in the price of oranges; their use may diminish markedly. The proportions of beef and of pork eaten by meat consumers will depend on their price; an increase in the price of pork will cause families to use more beef (if the price of beef doesn't increase at the same time). Economic conditions in a country will have a real effect on food selection. Prosperous people, able to buy a variety of foods, will use smaller quantities of cheap foods and larger amounts of expensive foods. The reverse situation, of course, occurs also. In a period of economic depression in North America people use less meat and eggs and eat more bread. Some years ago it was observed in Great Britain that the amount of fat which people obtained from food depended on their financial circumstances; high-income persons ate more fat than did low-income people. This relation of fat intake to economic circumstances holds true for various countries. North Americans consume a great deal more fat than do the citizens of Japan. It is said that the standard of living in the United States and in Canada has been elevated considerably in the past fifty years (or is it just that we have more gadgets?). During that period there has been a substantial reduction in the use of bread and of cereal products. At the same time there has been an increase in the use of milk, fruits, vegetables, and eggs.

It has been shown that food-buying habits can be changed by example or by education. If children are given a good noon meal at school and become acquainted with foods new to them, there will be a carry-over to the home. A great deal of information and advice has been given to the public in recent years. Quite often it is difficult or impossible to demonstrate that advice about food selection has had an effect. So many factors influence food choice, as we have already seen.

A good deal of money could be safely bet on the truth of the statement that many people, asked why they eat particular foods, would answer, "Because I like them." This is an important factor influencing food choice. Of course, fondness or liking for individual foods can change, or be changed by familiarity. Likes and dislikes of unfamiliar foods can be developed in children. The use of food as a punishment or as a reward can cause a child to dislike or like the food in question. We don't need to wonder why children like ice cream when it is given as a reward or as a special treat. The mother who says, "If you are a good boy, you can have a piece of candy," can expect the child to be fond of candy. Liking for unfamiliar foods can be encouraged in children by giving them a small portion of the new food and by increasing the size of the helping as familiarity develops. Life is a lot more interesting when we are willing to try new foods. A good deal of the fun of travel comes from trying new foods or new methods of cooking. A lot of people miss this pleasure. Recently, a well-known movie star was quoted as telling a reporter when she returned from Europe: "I don't want to go back—it was impossible to get good malted milks or hamburgers and there were no barbecues."

The food selection of most people depends on habits, many of which may have developed in childhood. People tend to be guided automatically by these habits. They like the foods to which they are accustomed. Most people either do not know, or do not care, that the body has certain requirements which must be satisfied by foods. If some of these requirements are not met, disease can develop. Our health depends on the satisfaction of these requirements. The intelligent way to select food is to know about the requirements and to know which foods we should use to meet the needs. There is a wide-spread impression that the selection of food on the health basis causes meals, and the eating of them, to be unpleasant and a kind of penance. That is, of course, not true. We can have very pleasant, attractive meals (just as tasty as our present ones) by selecting foods intelligently. We can accustom ourselves to the habit of eating foods on the health basis. Even more important, we can develop that kind of food habit in children.

# CHAPTER 3

# *The Choice of Foods
   for Health and Pleasure*

The food we eat must serve a number of purposes in the body if health is to be attained and maintained. One of the main difficulties is that most people don't know about the real needs, or, if they do know, they eat as if they didn't care. The needs are very simple to understand and they can be explained easily.

## A. *Growth*

Obviously, food is needed for growth. A house cannot be constructed without building material. Our bodies cannot grow unless the substances which form the body are supplied. No miracle is involved; the needed substances come from foods.

The hard framework of the body, the bones, contain a great deal of calcium and phosphorus. So do the teeth.

21

These two nutrients are required as soon as bones and teeth start to develop in the baby several months before birth. They are supplied to the baby by the mother who, in turn, must obtain them from foods eaten by her to prevent her own body being deprived of them. After the baby is born, calcium and phosphorus will continue to be supplied by the mother, if she breast-feeds her baby. As children grow, the increase in the size of the bones makes continued supplies of calcium and phosphorus necessary, if the bones are to be healthy. We might decide that the need for calcium and phosphorus would end when growth stops. This is not true. Calcium may not stay put in the bones even if it does in the teeth when they are fully formed. Calcium serves purposes other than the building of bone. A fairly constant amount of calcium is maintained in the blood and in all of the fluids of the body since calcium in the blood is essential for blood-clotting. Calcium in fluids bathing the nerves has a marked effect on the activity of the nerves. If we do not take enough calcium in food, it is withdrawn from bone to keep the amount in the blood constant. To add to the need for calcium, a small amount is lost every day in urine and in feces. What this all adds up to, is that an intake of calcium is needed throughout life to keep the body from developing a deficit. Of course, the need is greatest when growth is taking place. The greatest need for calcium is in adolescence, since bones increase markedly in size during teen-age growth. Like calcium, phosphorus serves purposes other than bone formation; it is needed to help move fat around the body and for the utilization of carbohydrate (starch and sugar). As in the case of calcium, some phosphorus is being lost every day; there is need for a continuous intake throughout life.

Those of us who are not engineers regard with great admiration and respect the construction of a large building. The work seems so complicated that we wonder how it is done without mistakes. The formation of bone is a complicated business also. A variety of substances is needed for both large buildings and for bones. At least two of the vitamins are necessary for the formation of really healthy bones. In the case of any nutrient, we must be concerned not only with the quantity in the meals we eat, but also with the amount absorbed and used in the body. The absorption of calcium and of phosphorus may not be particularly efficient. Sometimes people absorb only about one-fifth of the calcium in eaten food. Vitamin D has a very beneficial effect on the absorption of calcium and may cause the amount absorbed to double. Of course, this makes more calcium available for building into bones and teeth. Another matter of concern is whether the incorporation of calcium into bones and teeth goes on normally, producing healthy structures. Both vitamins C and D help the building of bones and teeth. It follows that we should be sure that ample supplies of these vitamins are available during growth. Any wise father or mother would wish children to have healthy, properly formed, bones and teeth. To ensure this, it is necessary to guide children to eat the foods which supply calcium, phosphorus, vitamin C, and to ensure an adequate supply of vitamin D. Practical ways of ensuring such supplies will be described later.

The soft parts of the body (muscles, liver, heart, and so on) contain a great deal of water. Muscle contains water to the extent of three-quarters of the total weight. Blood and other fluids in the body contain a high proportion of water. Ordinarily, people don't think much about the need for water unless they have to do without it, or with very little. Then it is realized how important water is. We can live for a much longer period without solid food than we can survive without water. A man of average weight needs two to three quarts of water a day. The amount needed depends on how hard he works, climatic temperatures, and how well kidneys are functioning.

Next to water, the chief constituent of the soft parts of the body are substances belonging to a group called protein (this word means "of first importance"). There is a great variety of proteins in the body, and in food. They are grouped together because they are formed from simpler units called amino acids. There are nineteen of these amino acids, and proteins differ from each other in the assortment and the quantities of the different amino acids. If this sounds complicated, think of building brick walls with nineteen kinds of bricks available. One wall could contain all nineteen different bricks in certain proportions, another might be built from different proportions of the nineteen bricks and would look entirely different from the first wall. A third wall could be constructed with fifteen kinds of bricks. We could build many different walls using varying assortments of nineteen kinds of brick. There may be fifty different proteins in the foods we eat. During digestion the food proteins are broken down to the amino acids and these are absorbed. The body uses these absorbed amino acids to build a variety of different proteins to serve special purposes. There is a catch in this building of proteins in the body. Eight of the amino acids must be available and must be supplied by food, if the body is to remain healthy. The body gets along without a food supply of the other eleven amino acids because they can be produced in the body. Obviously, proteins are required for growth and an adequate supply of the proteins which will furnish the essential amino acids is all-important during growth. The protein supply situation is further complicated because the proteins in our body do not stay put. The body proteins are constantly wearing away and there must be a continuous new supply (particularly of the essential amino acids) throughout life.

Food proteins which contain all the essential amino acids are called complete—that is an easily understood name, isn't it? Food proteins which lack some of the essential amino acids are called incomplete. The simplest way to obtain a supply of all of the essential amino acids is to select foods which contain complete proteins. Animal-source foods like meat, fowl, fish, eggs, milk, cheese, contain complete proteins. Proteins in grains and in vegetables are incomplete.

While the simplest way of obtaining all the essential amino acids is to eat foods which contain complete proteins, we can get the same result by eating a variety of foods with incomplete proteins. The essential amino acid missing in one food will be present in another food. If we do rely mainly on incomplete protein-foods, we have to use a larger total amount of protein. Vegetarians can get all the essential amino acids without eating meat, fish, or fowl. In some countries this is necessary because these foods are not available. If meat, fish, or fowl are available, why be a vegetarian?

## B. *Energy*

Humans are warm-blooded animals living in a cold environment. It is necessary to keep the body warm to maintain life. Just like a radiator, the body is continuously losing heat to the surroundings (have you been in a crowded bus lately?). Actually, it is necessary to have the body temperature kept fairly constant. This is done by generating heat in the body and by controlling the heat loss by sweating. The evaporation of sweat increases heat loss and tends to keep the body from becoming too hot. Two hundred years ago it was taught that body heat was produced by the friction of the blood moving through the blood vessels. The famous French scientist, Lavoisier, demonstrated that heat was produced in the body by a chemical reaction (oxidation) between food substances and the oxygen from the atmosphere. His observations clearly settled the function of food in providing heat in the body.

To maintain life, energy is expended for more than heat production. The beating of the heart, the work of the lungs in breathing, the activities of other vital organs, all expend energy. Like heat production, the energy for the vital functions is produced in the body by the oxidation of food substances.

When exercise or physical work is done (if we can't help it), energy is expanded. Again, this energy is provided by the oxidation of food substances. The amount of energy depends on the severity of the exercise or work. If a person sits most of the time, the amount of energy used in work is only a fraction of the total energy need of his body.

Since a great deal of the energy produced in the body

is used for heat, it is reasonable that the energy production should be measured in heat units. The unit used is the calorie and it is the amount of heat required to raise the temperature of one kilogram (2.2 lbs.) of water 1°C (1.8°F). This is the "large" calorie; the "small" calorie, not used in nutrition, is the amount of heat required to raise the temperature of one gram of water 1°C.

The energy values of foods are also expressed in calories. The constituents of foods which can be oxidized to provide energy are: carbohydrates (starch and sugar), fats, and proteins. Proteins are used as constituents of soft parts of the body and also to furnish energy. Equal weights of carbohydrates and of proteins have equal energy, or calorie, value. Similar weights of fats furnish twice as much energy as do carbohydrates or proteins. It is useful to remember that fats are concentrated sources of energy, especially if you wish to reduce your calorie intake.

Maintenance-energy needs (body heat plus vital organ activity) vary from person to person, and in the same person from time to time. Maintenance-energy needs vary with the size (or weight) and in adults they can be expressed as twelve to sixteen calories per pound of body weight. Sex has no effect on these maintenance needs, but women generally weigh less than men. Age does effect maintenance needs since they decrease as we become older; activity also lessens in most people as they grow older. During growth some of the food substances are used to increase the size of the body and hence cannot be used for energy. Per pound of weight the total calorie intake of children should be greater than for adults—especially so in adolescence.

## C. *Other Varied Needs*

Blood is normally red because it contains a red substance called hemoglobin. This substance in turn contains iron. Hemoglobin serves a truly essential function in carrying oxygen from the lungs to all parts of the body and in moving to the lungs carbon dioxide (a product of the oxidation of food substances) so that the carbon dioxide can be got rid of in expired air. Hemoglobin is continuously breaking down in the body and the loss must be made good; otherwise, an anemia will develop. To produce hemoglobin, iron must be available. Normally there is very little iron lost from the body unless there is a loss of blood. Men can get along for a fairly long time without an intake of iron, if storage of iron is good at the start, and if there is no hemorrhage. Women, between puberty and the menopause, lose sufficient blood during menstruation to make necessary an intake of iron.

The thyroid gland is in the neck, straddling the windpipe. This gland controls the rate of oxidation of food substances in the body. The control is brought about by a substance, the thyroid hormone, which is produced in the gland and circulated about the body. This thyroid hormone contains a constant amount of iodine and this nutrient should be available in adequate amounts to enable the thyroid gland to make the hormone. If the supply of iodine is insufficient, the gland tries to make up for the lack of iodine by increasing in size. This increase in size of the thyroid gland is called goiter. There are several kinds of goiter; the kind resulting from a lack of iodine is known as "simple goiter." Simple goiter can be prevented by making sure that the intake of iodine is adequate.

A series of vitamins is needed by humans, generally to serve purposes specific for each vitamin. It has been pointed out that vitamin D improves the absorption of calcium and its building into bones and teeth during growth. Nature did not intend us to obtain vitamin D from foods. When the skin is exposed to sunlight or to an artificial source of ultraviolet light, two substances ordinarily present in the skin are converted into vitamin D, which then is available to increase the absorption and utilization of calcium. In winter months in temperate and cold climates, the amount of sunlight is reduced and clothing reduces the amount of skin exposed to sunlight. This lessens still further the formation of vitamin D. In many cities the amount of ultraviolet reaching the skin from sunlight is reduced by the smoke and dirt in the air. Under these circumstances an external supply of vitamin D is needed in persons in whom growth is taking place. The oil from cod, halibut, and some other fish livers is an excellent source of vitamin D. This vitamin can be made industrially and concentrated products are readily available. The strength of vitamin D preparations is expressed in units.

Some seven or eight vitamins are definitely needed by humans to preserve health. Originally, these were named by using letters of the alphabet. In some cases, the letters are still used. For some of the vitamins more explicit names, based on chemical composition, are now in use. Such names will be used here because they are becoming familiar, even to children. The proper name for vitamin C is ascorbic acid. As has been noted earlier, this vitamin helps the building of calcium into teeth and bones and is very much needed during growth. However, this vitamin serves other, and quite different, purposes. It helps to keep the walls of the small blood vessels (the capillaries) in a firm, healthy state. When insufficient ascorbic acid is available, the walls of the capillaries are weakened and rupture easily, allowing blood to escape. The hemorrhages thus produced are characteristic of the disease, scurvy, which is caused by a deficiency of ascorbic acid. It has been known for over two hundred years that scurvy can be prevented by using fresh fruits and vegetables (or fruit juices). Under most modern circumstances, adults in North America do not develop scurvy, but in some cities in the past few years a number of babies have had scurvy because their mothers did not give them orange juice.

Vitamin A, for some years, was referred to as the growth vitamin and some people called it the anti-infective vitamin. Neither term was accurate. All essential food constituents are necessary for growth and, in this respect, vitamin A is no more valuable than complete proteins, or calcium, or most of the other vitamins. If we fail to take in any essential nutrient in needed amounts, it is likely that our resistance to infection will be lessened. In this respect, also, vitamin A is no more valuable than any other essential nutrient. However, this vitamin does serve at least two real functions in humans. In the back part of the eye there is a substance called visual purple. This substance consists of vitamin A linked to a special protein. During the process of vision, visual purple is used up. The supply can be replaced if vitamin A is available. If there is not enough vitamin A on hand, the quantity of visual purple needed for full vision cannot be maintained. This situation shows up, particularly, when people are exposed to bright light (as on a clear, sunny day) and a great deal of visual purple is used. In the subdued light of evening, vision may be badly affected. This is called night-blindness. It should be noted that night-blindness can be produced by an abnormality in the structure of the eye; not all night-blindness is due to a lack of vitamin A. This vitamin is connected with another eye disease, one given the complicated name, xerophthalmia. In this disease skin surfaces about the eye are weakened by a lack of vitaman A and an infection may get established in the weakened skin. If that is the case, blindness can be produced. This disease occurred in children living in areas where the supply of vitamin A was meager. Some foods contain vitamin A and others contain a substance, carotene, which can be turned into vitamin A in the body. Either source is satisfactory.

A group of vitamins, frequently called the B complex, contains a number of different substances. At least three of these are needed by humans and it is guessed that several others may be essential, also. The three known to be required are thiamine, riboflavin, and nicotinic acid (or niacin). These vitamins are quite different from each other in composition and they serve distinct functions in the body. The oxidation of carbohydrates, fats, and proteins is brought about in the body, not in one stroke, but by complicated, step-wise processes. The B vitamins are accelerators for particular steps in the complicated oxidative processes. Thiamine is an interesting case; it helps at one step in the utilization of carbohydrate. If thiamine is lacking, this step is prevented and the utilization of carbohydrate cannot go on by normal processes. Naturally, this failure has a marked effect in the body and there develops a disease known as beriberi. There are two types of beriberi. In the dry form the legs become paralyzed and walking is difficult and finally impossible. In wet beriberi an accumulation of water causes swelling and puffiness. This disease is hardly ever seen in the United States, in Canada, or in other highly developed countries. It has been far too prevalent in Eastern areas where food is scarce.

Like thiamine, riboflavin and niacin serve in expediting oxidative processes. It is not clear how much harm is caused by a deficiency of riboflavin, but a long-standing lack of niacin produces pellagra. Pellagra, in the period between 1900 and 1940, was a very serious problem in the Southern states. Pellagra is characterized by a rash on the portions of the skin exposed to sunlight. Diarrhea is commonly present. In severe pellagra mental conditions develop. The increased use of meat and other foods supplying niacin, owing to an improvement in economic conditions, has caused the almost complete disappearance of pellagra. The disease still occurs in other parts of the world and it could reappear in North America if care is not taken.

There are several important points to remember about the vitamins. A prolonged failure to obtain adequate intake of many of them will cause deficiency diseases. However, the really important thing about the vitamins is that they are required for *normal* functions in the body and are essential for health. This does not mean that intakes in excess of healthful amounts will produce a super kind of health or abnormal resistance to colds or other infections. If we take excess amounts of ascorbic acid, of thiamine, of riboflavin, or of niacin we will not have super health but we will enrich the sewage because the excess amounts will be excreted in the urine. Excess intakes of vitamins A and D are not got rid of but accumulate in the body. Very large intakes of these two vitamins will cause damage and are not only not beneficial but are harmful. Massive doses of vitamin D will not prevent colds or cure arthritis. In prosperous countries, adequate supplies of all the vitamins except vitamin D can be easily obtained from foods. In later chapters, the dependable food sources of vitamins and of other nutrients will be described. It pays to eat wisely and not waste money on pills.

CHAPTER | 4

## The Dairy Foods: Milk, Cheese, Butter

One of the advantages of living in one of the prosperous countries is the general—and generous—availability of milk, cheese, and butter (or margarine). The advantage is not always appreciated, nor do we realize the marked improvement in the safety and in the distribution of these foods in the past fifty years. When I was a youngster in a small Canadian city, milk was delivered to our home by the farmer who owned the cows. He brought a can to the back door and measured out the desired amount into a pitcher. The milk was cheap, in comparison to present prices, but it was not safe to drink. No one in our family contracted tuberculosis or undulant fever, but we could have. At that time, certified or pasteurized milk were both unheard of in our area. Now, no milk may be sold in all Ontario (an area larger than Texas) unless it has been properly pasteurized. This process, in which bacteria in milk are killed by heating milk to a suitable temperature, causes milk to be safe when it is obtained by the household. Pasteurization does *not* harm milk and it should be compulsory everywhere—even in farm households. I would prefer to do without milk rather than run the risk of a milk-carried infection.

## Milk

In the United States, in Canada, and wherever available, milk is a valuable and economical food. Milk contains a complete, high-value protein. Two quarts of milk contain the same amount of protein as does one pound of average beef. Use this information to do a bit of simple arithmetic. Compare the cost of protein from milk and beef in your own area. When that is done, remember that protein is needed at any age. Milk is an excellent source of protein for older people, who may not get enough if they stop eating meat because of chewing difficulties.

Protein is not the only reason for using milk. It is our most convenient, excellent source of calcium for day-to-day use. If we exclude milk, and eat little cheese, our supply of calcium will be low. This is just as true for adults as it is for children. Expectant mothers should have a liberal supply of calcium during the last third of pregnancy to make sure that the baby's bones and teeth are properly formed. The easiest way to get a liberal intake of calcium is to drink milk. Sometimes, pregnant women are advised to take tablets of calcium gluconate. Milk is a cheaper source of calcium and also supplies protein needed for the growth of the baby.

Milk is an excellent source of the vitamin, riboflavin. There is a resemblance to the situation regarding cal-

cium. Only one other food is a top-grade source of
riboflavin; that food is liver. Many people find it easier
to drink milk than to eat liver.

To add to the three nutrition reasons for using milk,
it should be noted that it is an easily digested food, suitable even for "delicate" stomachs (whatever they are).

You may have heard the statement that "milk is a
perfect food." That is *not* true. Raw milk contains a
small amount of ascorbic acid which is destroyed by
pasteurization, but even raw milk is not a good source
of ascorbic acid. Milk contains very little iron. It is
not a good source of niacin. Milk is a convenient, economical and very useful source of high-quality protein, of
calcium, and of riboflavin. Those three constituents
make milk an important food which should not be
neglected.

Should skim milk be used? Yes, if you are concerned
with keeping down your weight. Cup for cup, skim milk
has about half the calorie value of whole milk. Cup for
cup, skim milk supplies the same amounts of protein, of
riboflavin, and of calcium as does whole milk. The use
of skim milk may save money, also. Removal of fat from
milk, however, lowers the amount of vitamin A because
that vitamin is dissolved in the fat. Don't worry about
that; vitamin A can be obtained more cheaply by eating
a number of vegetables.

Dry skim milk is a very economical method of providing the values of fresh milk. Made up with the right
amount of water, the reconstituted skim milk, cup for
cup, supplies as much protein, riboflavin, and calcium as
does fresh, whole milk and is much cheaper. If your
family doesn't like the taste of milk made from dry skim
milk, try letting it stand in the refrigerator eight to ten

hours before use. Another expedient to save money is to mix reconstituted skim milk in equal amounts with fresh whole milk. Dry skim milk is excellent for cooking.

The milk from different animals is not entirely the same. But for all practical purposes it doesn't matter whether we use milk from cows, goats, or buffaloes (if we are in India). The fat in goats' milk is present in very small droplets which do not separate out, and this makes goats' milk easily digestable. Human milk does not have the same composition as cows' milk. Breast milk was designed to nourish the human baby. It is true that cows' milk can be modified by adding water and sugar. The best food for the human infant—and the safest—is breast milk. If the sight of a mother feeding her baby were not taboo in our best circles, or if some young mothers were not so selfish, babies would be a great deal better fed.

How much milk should we use? The following quantities are the least which should be used, *every day*, to ensure suitable intakes of protein, of calcium, and of riboflavin:

Children, up to about 12 years: at least 1 pint.
Adolescents: at least 1½ pints (more calcium is needed).
Adults of any age: at least ½ pint.
Expectant mothers: at least 1½ pints during the second
        half of pregnancy.

The frequently used slogan, "a quart of milk a day" is a bad one which should not be repeated. Young children can be given too much milk. When that happens, children are unlikely to eat suitable amounts of other needed foods. A child of five or six cannot hold a quart of milk a day *and* other necessary foods.

There are some silly notions about milk. Pasteurized milk is a safe and very useful food. It does not cause phlegm in the throat. It does not cause cancer. It is a valuable food at any age and not just for children. It is important to start the habit of drinking milk in childhood and to continue it as long as life lasts.

## Cheese

Essentially, cheese is the protein from milk. However, most of the calcium remains with the protein, except in cottage cheese, which is low in calcium. An appreciable portion of riboflavin from milk is present in cheese—but not the full amount.

There are many different kinds of cheese. Cheddar cheese is a commonly available one, widely made and used in the United States and in Canada. Cheddar cheese may be ripened or cured by storage. Such "old" cheese can have a most satisfying flavor, at least for older people. Cheddar cheese is generally an economical source of protein and of calcium—one ounce of Cheddar cheese furnishes about the same amount of calcium as do six ounces of milk.

While Cheddar cheese is the main kind used in the United States and in Canada, a number of varieties have become popular. Some of these were imported originally from Europe. Roquefort, Camembert, Edam, and Swiss cheeses were in the luxury class. These kinds of cheeses are now made in North America. Some cheeses are altered in flavor and appearance by allowing particular bacteria to grow and even produce mold. Roquefort, Blue, Camembert, are of this type. If you are not a connoisseur of cheese, you may never have tried some of these varieties. If you are a connoisseur of cheese, I hail you as a kindred spirit. I feel sorry for the people who don't like cheese. By itself, cheese is a grand food. Think what a generous piece of old Cheddar will do for even homemade apple pie (the pie should be warm, shouldn't it?). Netherlanders may be accustomed to having cheese for breakfast. That sounds like a queer custom until it's tried. An addition of cheese can do a great deal for a number of foods by improving both taste and nutritive value. Macaroni with plenty of good cheese is tasty, cheap and nutritious. What would spaghetti, or even onion soup, be without cheese?

There are a number of different kinds of processed cheese and cheese spreads. In general these are not economical because they contain more water than does Cheddar. A true lover of cheese would not use them because of flavor.

It is a very good plan to use at least three ounces of cheese a week to increase supplies of protein and of calcium and to have a really tasty food or food combination.

I feel particularly sorry for the people who are convinced that cheese should not be eaten because it is constipating or because it is indigestible. Neither statement is true; both are old wives' tales.

### Butter (or Margarine)

People who eat bread do not usually like it without a spread on it. The two spreads commonly used are butter and margarine. Since they are largely fat they do add calories. If you are interested in weight control you will cut down on bread anyway.

Except from the viewpoint of calorie contributions there is no proved harm from eating butter or margarine. In the past few years there has been a great deal said about fat intake in relation to heart disease. As we shall see in Chapter 14, there is no certain evidence to prove that there is a relation between heart disease and fat intake.

For some years there was a great disturbance, mostly political, about margarine. Dairy people opposed the sale of margarine, for reasons which are quite obvious: margarine can be made and sold at prices generally much lower than can butter. The early kinds of margarine were not satisfactory from the viewpoints of taste or of nutritive value. Both situations have been cleared up. Modern margarine is a satisfactory food and is useful for families who cannot afford butter. Butter contains vitamin A, but the amount is variable. This vitamin is now added to margarine so that it is at least equal to butter as a source of vitamin A. For some time it was claimed that margarine is not digested as easily and is absorbed less completely than butter. From the aspects of digestibility and absorbability, butter and margarine are equal. If it is wrong to color margarine it is wrong, also, to add color to butter (a common practice). The controversy about margarine has now largely disappeared. It is unlikely in the future that professors in state-supported colleges or staff members in experiment stations will be dismissed for daring to state that margarine is a satisfactory food.

CHAPTER | **5**

# *Fruits*

A high school student in our city told a teacher of physical and health education that the reason for eating oranges for breakfast was to counteract the taste left in the mouth from the previous night. That could be an advantage for some people but it is not the main reason for eating fruit or drinking fruit juice. The real reason was established in 1734 by James Lind, a surgeon in the British Navy. Lind was concerned with the cause and the prevention of scurvy, a disease then common among crews of ships on long voyages. Lind showed that scurvy could be prevented by using juice from citrus fruit or by eating fruits and vegetables. The prevention of scurvy in babies is still important but everyone needs the vitamin known as ascorbic acid, supplied by many fruits and vegetables.

Not all fruits are equally good sources of ascorbic acid. The really dependable sources are oranges and grapefruit or their juices. The simplest way to ensure a decent intake of ascorbic acid is to have a medium-size orange, or half a grapefruit, or four ounces of orange or grapefruit juice every morning with breakfast. The fruit or fruit juice does taste pretty good; maybe the high school student had a valid reason.

Some other fruits are excellent sources of ascorbic acid, also. Strawberries are a good example. An average serving of fresh or frozen strawberries will supply about as much ascorbic acid as will a medium-size orange. Cantaloupes are another excellent source.

Some fruits are poor sources of ascorbic acid: peaches, pears, and popular varieties of apples. Apple juice contains little ascorbic acid. However, ascorbic acid can be cheaply produced commercially and can be added to apple juice during processing.

Several popular fruits are in-between excellent and poor, as suppliers of ascorbic acid. Such fruits as limes, tangerines, pineapples, watermelons, come into this category. Of course, there is a simple method of getting a greater amount of ascorbic acid if we are using such fruits, and that is to eat more.

Ascorbic acid can be lost to a greater extent during cooking than can any other food constituent. This vitamin is soluble in water and can be extracted from food which is cooked in water. Moreover, ascorbic acid is oxidized easily (a chemical reaction between ascorbic acid and oxygen takes place and this chemical reaction destroys ascorbic acid). The oxidation of ascorbic acid can take place at room temperature but it is increased by heat. The loss of ascorbic acid during cooking can be decreased by some easy-to-use precautions which will be discussed in connection with vegetables (next chapter).

Of course, the most ascorbic acid can be obtained if the food containing it is not cooked. This is one of the two reasons why it is useful to use oranges and grapefruit regularly. They are not usually cooked. Some people liked baked oranges and baked grapefruit. Those fruits are so good, as is, that any cooking is unnecessary and unwise.

What about canned juice or concentrated juice? During the process of concentrating juice or of sterilization, a great deal of the natural ascorbic acid may be destroyed. Commercially produced ascorbic acid is available readily and can be added to make good the loss. This is now common practice, and canned citrus juice and concentrated juice are practically always dependable products.

There is a question about the retention of ascorbic acid in citrus juice left over and saved for use later. If the juice is kept in a refrigerator, preferably in a closed container, no loss will occur within at least twenty-four hours, and the juice is likely to be satisfactory for two or three days, if it is kept cold.

The habit of having citrus fruit, or juice, for breakfast has spread widely in recent years and people do get the impression that breakfast is the only suitable time. It doesn't matter what time of the day we use citrus fruit to be sure of a supply of ascorbic acid. It is just as good for dessert at any meal or even in the evening. Citrus juice is refreshing at any time of the day, especially in hot weather.

There is a very good reason for thinking about fruit for dessert, particularly for people who wish to reduce or to keep from gaining weight. Practically all fruits have low calorie values and give a pleasant ending to a meal.

A fruit salad is low in calories unless it is smothered with whipped cream.

In several cities in North America in the past few years an undue number of babies have developed scurvy. Human milk contains ascorbic acid and the amount supplied by breast milk is generally sufficient to prevent scurvy in the baby. Feeding formulas made from cows' milk will not contain sufficient ascorbic acid to prevent scurvy, and babies fed such formulas need a special supply of ascorbic acid. The easiest and the most sensible way is to give the baby orange juice, and the amount necessary to prevent scurvy is two ounces a day. Most babies tolerate orange juice without trouble if it is started slowly in small amounts. The orange juice habit is a good one to start because it is one which should be continued through life. Ascorbic acid can be obtained in tablets or in various vitamin products. It seems silly to start a baby on a habit of obtaining this essential vitamin from vitamin products when it is easily obtainable from foods. It is much better to start habits which can and which should be continued to old age.

Many fruits have values in addition to ascorbic acid. Fruits are likely to contain cellulose. This substance is a complicated relative of starch. Unlike starch, cellulose cannot be digested by humans. Since cellulose is not digested, it supplies bulk in the intestines. Hence fruits, and vegetables, which contain cellulose have a laxative effect. This is another good reason for the generous use of fruits, especially by older people.

Fruits, particularly acid ones, have an additional virtue not commonly realized and which some people refuse to believe. There is a notion that acid fruits like oranges and grapefruit increase the amount of acid in the body.

The actual effect is the opposite to this notion. In the body, the fruit acids are converted to bases (the opposite of acids) and these bases neutralize acids from other sources. It is likely that you know elderly people who will not eat oranges or grapefruit because they are sure that the acid in the fruit increases the amount of acid in the body and consequently will either cause rheumatism or make it worse. Rheumatism, or arthritis, is not caused by the use of any particular food; it cannot be prevented or cured by using or refraining from eating any particular food.

There is yet another notion about acid fruits. This notion is that we cannot drink milk in the same meal with acid fruits because the acid from the fruit will curdle the milk. The digestive juice, normally found in the stomach, is more acid than any fruit or fruit juice, and the acidity in the stomach juice is necessary for the part of digestion which takes place in the stomach. Incidentally, the acid in the stomach juice curdles the milk and that is an aid to the digestion of the protein in milk. There are a lot of very foolish notions about foods. We should attempt to get reliable information and not believe the notions.

# CHAPTER | 6

## *Vegetables*

One of the real delights in a modern supermarket is the wide variety of fresh, frozen, and canned vegetables. It is a great pleasure to look at all the different vegetables. They are very nice to look at and they do add interest and health properties to meals—if they are used. One of the bad features of life is the rigidity of the habits we began to form in childhood. Some of us grew up at a time and in areas where only potatoes and a few other vegetables were available from late October until the next summer. We became accustomed to eating only those few vegetables and we do not want to try vegetables which are new to us. We miss a great deal of pleasure. What is just as important, we deprive ourselves of the healthful values of the vegetables which we will not try.

In refusing to eat unaccustomed vegetables men are generally worse than women. In our city the various men's service clubs have very similar menus for luncheons. The vegetables can be predicted in advance: potatoes and peas, or occasionally green beans. The reason for this monotony of vegetables is that most men will not eat any others. It's easy to trace this self-imposed restriction back to childhood. In a school lunchroom beets were served one day. Most of the children, having been brought up in an approved modern manner to express themselves, threw the beets on the floor as a protest against the effrontery of serving a new vegetable. That tells a great deal about home conditions, doesn't it?

Vitamin A is needed by babies, children, and adults. We can obtain vitamin A from whole milk, from butter or margarine, and in generous amounts from liver. Vegetables do not contain vitamin A but they do contain a related substance known as carotene. This carotene is yellow-orange and is responsible for the color of carrots, of squash and of most yellow vegetables. Carotene is also present in green vegetables, but we are not aware of it in those vegetables because the color of the carotene is masked by green. Carotene can be changed into vitamin A in the body after it is absorbed. This way of obtaining vitamin A is important and useful because most of the vegetables which contain a lot of carotene are generally cheap. It is more economical to use these vegetables and get needed vitamin A by converting the carotene into the vitamin than it is to buy the vitamin already formed in animal-source foods.

Some vegetables will furnish us, in one average portion, sufficient carotene to give the vitamin A needed for a day. These vegetables are: carrots, collards, kale, squash, turnip greens, sweet potatoes, and yams. Do you notice two types in this list, yellow (carrots, squash, sweet potatoes, yams), and green-leafed (collards, kale, turnip greens)? You may have heard the advice to use yellow and green-leafed vegetables frequently. The reason for the advice is the carotene content. Unfortunately, not all green vegetables are valuable in this respect. Asparagus, peas, cabbage, tomatoes, are only moderately good with respect to carotene. This doesn't mean that these vegetables are not worth eating.

To go back to fruit for a moment, there is one fruit which contains a large amount of carotene. That fruit, dried apricots, could be guessed because of its color.

A number of vegetables contain generous amounts of ascorbic acid. Here is a list of some which are particularly useful in supplying ascorbic acid: asparagus, broccoli, Brussels sprouts, cabbage, collards, green peppers, spinach, turnip greens. In this list, green-leafed vegetables are predominant. This is another sound reason for the advice about using yellow and green-leafed vegetables frequently. If you cannot or will not use citrus fruits, sufficient ascorbic acid can be obtained from vegetables, if the vegetables are sensibly selected and properly cooked.

Several other vegetables are moderately good in supplying ascorbic acid. Two of these are important because they are used frequently. These are potatoes and tomatoes. People who eat potatoes every day can get a good deal of ascorbic acid if care is taken with cooking. If we relied on tomato juice as the only source of ascorbic acid, it would be necessary to drink twice the quantity as of orange or grapefruit juice. Some other vegetables which are moderately good sources of ascorbic acid are: beans (snap or string), beets, parsnips, peas, sauerkraut, sweet potatoes, turnips.

In connection with vegetables giving ascorbic acid, it

is essential to remember that this vitamin can be extracted from the vegetables into cooking water, that it can be destroyed by oxidation, and that this oxidation is stepped up by heat. Losses of ascorbic acid from vegetables can be reduced by a few precautions:

1. Obviously, if a vegetable is not cooked, the loss of ascorbic acid will be almost nil. Raw cabbage makes an appetizing salad, liked by most people, and most of the ascorbic acid is retained. There will be a small loss since the exposure of cut surfaces to air at room temperature does bring about some oxidation; such loss will not be important during an hour or two.
2. The amount of extraction and the amount of oxidation varies with the amount of surface exposed to water or to air. The amount of surface can be kept down by leaving vegetables in the largest sized pieces that can be cooked.
3. The smaller the amount of water added for cooking, the smaller will be the extraction loss. It is better to bake vegetables than to boil them in water. Baked potatoes retain more ascorbic acid than do boiled or mashed potatoes.
4. If vegetables are allowed to stand after cooking and are kept warm, a great deal of oxidation goes on and there can be a really significant loss of ascorbic acid. The flavor deteriorates, too.
5. It is a distinct advantage to cook for the shortest period necessary to give an appetizing product.

Careful consideration of these precautions will show that procedures which reduce losses of ascorbic acid will give more appetizing results. Drowned, overcooked vegetables are not tasty for most people. Even the appearance suffers.

Some vegetables are useful as sources of other vitamins, in addition to vitamin A and ascorbic acid. Asparagus, collards, peas, potatoes, are moderately good foods in supplying thiamine and niacin. These vitamins, like ascorbic acid, are soluble in water and can be extracted by cooking water. The precautions suggested for the retention of ascorbic acid are useful for thiamine and niacin.

Some of you will remember Pop-Eye, who ate spinach to obtain iron. Spinach is not the only vegetable which is a good source of iron. Several other green-leafed vegetables supply as much iron as does spinach. Collards and turnip greens are two such vegetables. Cabbage and cauliflower are medium sources of iron.

There are at least two good health reasons for using generously a variety of vegetables. In general, yellow and green-leafed vegetables are valuable foods in giving carotene (to turn into vitamin A), ascorbic acid, and iron. Several other vegetables are useful sources of thiamine and niacin. These are not the only health reasons for using a variety of vegetables. Let us list a few more reasons. Some vegetables, like some fruits, contain appreciable cellulose and have a laxative effect. Potatoes are economical sources of energy—if you don't need to cut down your energy intake to lose weight. While it is true that the proteins in vegetables are incomplete, lacking some of the essential amino acids, bean protein is nearly as good as the protein in meat. People in northern China, who have used soya beans as a main item of food, have had a good reason for doing so. Beans are often described as meat alternates and can be used if meat is scarce, or if it is advisable to save money in buying food. New Englanders, brought up to eat baked beans, are using an economical source of fairly good protein.

A number of vegetables (not potatoes) have low energy values and can be used in generous amounts when weight reduction is desired. Green-leafed vegetables, with so many other virtues, have low calorie values. The cellulose which they contain supplies bulk. We can eat a lot of these vegetables, without having too much effect on energy intake and on weight.

If you are bored with this discussion of the healthful properties of vegetables, let's get back to thinking about their pleasurable character. The variety of colors makes meals look more appealing and attractive. A plateful of food does not need to look drab. That may seem to be a poor reason for eating vegetables. There are better reasons. Vegetables have a variety of flavors and they can be cooked in a variety of ways. Vegetables can be used to make meals more interesting, more appetizing, and less monotonous. Boiled carrots are all right, but carrots do not need to be always boiled. Even if they are boiled they can be served with a nice sauce. Baked carrots are attractive in appearance and in flavor.

This is getting close to the troublesome point about vegetables. Most men, and, indeed, many women are stick-in-the-muds when it comes to trying unfamiliar vegetables. They do lose a lot of pleasure. This writer is strongly in favor of healthful *and* interesting meals. One dodge helpful in getting the family to try a new vegetable is to serve small portions along with a well-accepted food. This works pretty well with children—of any age. Parents should do all they can to accustom children to a variety of foods. A variety is more likely to give all the health values, and a variety does make life more interesting. Of course, parents know that example has a good effect, if the example is sensible. Example can have a bad effect if father refuses to try a different vegetable and ridicules it. If kale cost you your first husband, cheer up. Maybe the second will eat kale.

# CHAPTER 7

# *Meat, Fish, Fowl, and Eggs*

Meat is probably the most generally used and the most popular food so far as most people in the United States, in Canada, and in other "have" countries are concerned. At present, people in many other areas are vegetarians, or nearly so, because they are compelled to be by a combination of scarce supplies and economic circumstances. In a few countries meat is not eaten because of religious reasons. Over a period of years many prominent persons have been vegetarians for humanitarian reasons; George Bernard Shaw was an interesting example. It was reported that Hitler was a vegetarian; if that was true, it could hardly have been for humanitarian reasons. Unless compelled to do without meat when it is not available or when it cannot be afforded, most people like meat and eat it generously.

Over a period of some years two entirely opposite questions have arisen regarding the eating of meat. It has

53

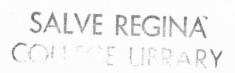

been claimed that meat has harmful effects (some present-day vegetarians say so). The opposite contention is that meat should be eaten generously and that we might be better off if we lived on meat alone, refraining from eating vegetables and cereal products. These two opposite arguments have been advanced for years and are still being advanced, vigorously so by a few people. Under the circumstances the only sensible thing to do is to consider the evidence, preferably that of a scientific and not hearsay nature.

The composition of various kinds of meat, of fish, and of fowl and the nutritive qualities of these foods are, in the main, very similar. True, there are some differences but they are insignificant in respect to whether or not these foods should be eaten and with regard to suitable amounts. For practical purposes we shall lump all of these foods together for the time being and refer to all of them as meat. In the next few paragraphs, this word will be used to cover various kinds of meat from animals, and fish and fowl will be included.

The two main constituents of meat are protein and fat. Water is, of course, also present but it will be ignored in the present discussion. Proportions of protein and fat vary from one kind of meat to another. An average figure for protein content is twenty per cent of the total weight, but the amount of protein in various kinds of meat may range from ten to twenty-eight or even thirty per cent. All the different proteins in meat are complete and of high-nutritive value with the exception of gelatin, which is an incomplete protein. The principal value of meat, in meeting nutrition needs, is in supplying high-quality protein. The proportion of fat in meat is highly variable. We tend to think of fat in meat in terms of what we see. In addition to the visible fat, there is likely to be considerable invisible fat, even in lean meat. Beef tongue has little or no visible fat yet it contains about twenty-three per cent fat. Lean beef liver has about sixteen per cent fat. The white meat of poultry contains comparatively little fat. Some commonly used fish have a low content of fat; others contain a great deal. Canned salmon may have ten to twenty per cent fat. The proportion of fat in lean meat has a considerable bearing on tenderness and palatability; meat low in fat is likely to have less appetite-appeal. In the past few years, people have been urged to use less fat because of the alleged, but unproved, effect of fat intake on the development of one or more kinds of heart disease. The increasing emphasis on the desirability of staying slim has induced many people to go easy on fat. For these reasons there have been developments in the production and use of meats having less fat. Time will tell whether these developments are a good idea.

It is obvious that meat is an excellent source of high-quality protein. Meat is, also, an excellent source of iron but it is a poor source of calcium. If we use milk and cheese in suitable amounts, we will not need to worry about meat not providing calcium. Some meats are excellent sources of vitamin A; this is true of liver. Muscle meats (the kind most often eaten) contain much less vitamin A. Practically all meat is a remarkably good source of thiamine and niacin. Liver contains considerable riboflavin; most other meat could not be classed as an excellent source of this vitamin.

In addition to a very popular palatability and excellent nutritive value, meat has at least one other virtue. Meat contains some substances which are soluble in water and which are easily extracted. These substances are called extractives. They help to give meat its distinctive flavor and they have another effect not always recognized. These extractives stimulate the flow of gastric juice and may increase appetite. Cubes made by concentrating beef extracts have been sold for many years. The impression used to be given that "beef tea" or bouillon made from these cubes was highly nutritious and excellent for invalids. It may contain some iron and some vitamins, but it is not a good way to obtain protein.

How much meat should people eat? A sensible recommendation is one average-sized serving of meat, fish, or fowl a day. This amount, along with suitable quantities of other good foods, will ensure sufficient protein, iron, and various vitamins. This amount is less than is currently used by a considerable number of people in the United States, in Canada, and in Britain. It is more than is available in many areas in Africa and in Asia.

Is a generous intake of meat harmful? Some of our vegetarian friends claim that the eating of meat has bad effects because it overworks the liver and kidneys. There is no scientific evidence that the liberal use of meat is harmful, at least in reasonably normal people. There is a large amount of evidence from human experience that the generous use of meat is not harmful.

Should we eat meat in very large amounts? Two main arguments are being used in attempts to have people eat larger amounts of meat. One argument has been advanced by Stefansson, the Arctic explorer, and it has been taken up by others. To put the contention in simple terms, it is stated that Eskimos under primitive conditions, before they were "ruined" by contact with white men, lived entirely on meat and fish and were remarkably healthy. The impression is given, perhaps unintentionally, that the Eskimos had sufficient sense to decide to live on meat and fish of their own accord. I have not yet seen it made clear that the Eskimos *had* to live on meat and fish; they couldn't help themselves. Just try to grow wheat, or apples, or potatoes in the Arctic. There weren't any supermarkets, even in driving distance. The question can be asked, but of course not answered, what sort of meals would primitive Eskimos have had, if foods other than meat and fish had been available? A partial answer can be attempted because, now that the Eskimos have been "ruined," they are using other foods. The claim is made that the level of health has markedly deteriorated. Unfortunately, there is very little sound information available about the health of Eskimos of fifty years ago. One point seems fairly clear: Eskimo men lived a very hazardous life and were likely to die fairly early in life because of accidents. Apparently, Eskimo women were likely to live much longer because life for them was much less hazardous. The claim is made that men who have tried living on meat alone while remaining in "civilized" areas remained in health, or even showed improved health. There is evidence, however, that attempts to maintain soldiers on meat alone had to be stopped within a short time because of adverse effects. One thing is clear: most of us cannot afford, financially, to live on meat as the only food. It's much too expensive.

Another contention about the generous use of meat involves the fat content and other food fats. This contention is that a very substantial increase in the use of meat and other fats is a good way to lose weight. This contention will be discussed in Chapter 12. One aspect can be pointed out: it is likely that people who have a very large proportion of fat in their meals may eat less food. Despite the high energy value of fat, the reduction in food intake may be so great that the calorie intake is decreased with a consequent loss in weight.

One of the problems related to the amount of meat which should be eaten is the high cost of meat. When there is a limited amount of money available for food, and for other necessities, it is advisable to get the most value possible. From the viewpoint of personal pleasure and of current habits, many people tend to spend a lot of money on meat, leaving less than suitable amounts for buying other foods. From the aspect of health, a variety of foods is advisable. When money is scarce, people should not spend more than one-fifth of the total food budget on meat, fish, and fowl. They should spend as much for milk and cheese as for meat, fish, and fowl, and an equal proportion should be used for the purchase of fruit and vegetables. This is not an argument for vegetarianism; it is intended as an argument for sensible food purchasing.

The major reason for the expensiveness of meat (excluding fish) is not the profit made by the cattle-raiser, or by the meat-packing industry, or by the butcher. Beef, pork, mutton, and poultry can never be produced cheaply because the production of meat is wasteful and expensive. Only about ten per cent of the food value of grain fed to meat-yielding animals is present in the meat as finally eaten by humans. If the grain were eaten directly, the human consumer would receive all of the grain's value. The high cost of meat can be explained in another way: if land is used to produce grain or vegetables to serve directly as human food, about eight times as much can be produced as when the crops are fed to animals to yield meat for human consumption. The high standard of living, with plenty of meat, is a wasteful business in so far as land is concerned. It's no wonder that meat is an expensive food.

In Britain, in most parts of the United States, and in Canada beef is generally the most popular meat. The proportion of beef to pork depends to a considerable extent on prices. In the United States and in Canada mutton is not popular; it is used to a much greater extent in several other countries. Chicken and turkey were eaten some years ago on festive occasions. The eating of chicken and turkey has become much more general in recent years. While the various kinds of meat, of fish, and of poultry can be grouped together for a general discussion of their value, there are some separate characteristics which should be mentioned:

*Beef and veal:* Veal is the meat from young calves; by law calves may not be slaughtered for use as meat until they are over three weeks old. There is an old story that veal is not as digestible as mature beef, but there is no evidence to support the notion. Baby beef from yearling cattle (about one year old) has become popular recently. Lean veal or beef is a very satisfactory source of protein.

*Pork:* While a considerable amount of fresh pork is used as chops or roasts, there is a larger consumption of cured ham and bacon. Pork differs from beef in having a greater proportion of fat scattered through the lean; for this reason pork is said to be less digestible than beef. This is probably true for people who have difficulty with fatty foods. Many of us can eat pork without difficulty, provided it is well cooked. Pork is noteworthy for containing a large amount of thiamine. Two pork chops will supply sufficient thiamine to meet the day's need of an average man.

*Mutton and lamb:* Lamb will be eaten with relish by many people in the United States and in Canada but they will refuse mutton. This is largely a question of habit. In other countries mutton is regarded as highly desirable meat. In nutritive value it resembles beef.

*Poultry:* The quality of the protein in poultry is as good as that in beef or pork. The contributions of iron and of vitamins are also about the same. White meat of chicken and of turkey is low in fat. There is a notion that dark meat may be harmful to people who may have either arthritis or gout. This is another notion that cannot be substantiated. The only real reason for a choice of white or dark meat is a matter of personal choice or habit. In recent years chickens have been raised by mass production methods and have become about as economical as most beef.

*Fish:* Modern methods of quick-freezing and of treatment with an antibiotic substance to prevent bacterial spoilage along with modern methods of shipping, have enabled us to enjoy fish the year round and in areas far removed from lakes or ocean. Canned salmon, canned tuna, and canned sardines are generally popular. Fish is just as good as beef or pork from the viewpoint of health values and is often cheaper. Good quality crab-meat and shrimps have become much more generally available and much more popular. They do add interesting variety to meals. Several other sea foods, like oysters and lobsters, are widely thought of as luxuries. They may be so from the standpoint of cost, but what delectable luxuries they are.

There was a remark above about the digestibility of pork. In general meats, fish, and fowl are thoroughly digested without difficulty by most people. Shortly after slaughter, beef is tough and not easily digested. If allowed to "hang," beef becomes more tender and more digestible. Cooking has an effect on the digestibility of meat. Rare beef is not as digestible as moderately done beef, and prolonged cooking can lessen digestibility. There can be some destruction of vitamins in meat during cooking; destruction is least when meat is cooked at high temperature for short periods. Roasting is likely to cause more destruction of the vitamin content than frying or broiling.

A problem frequently encountered in feeding older people is a meager intake of meat. Various reasons for the small intake of meat may exist. Some older people are convinced that meat is harmful. Dentures which fitted nicely when they were made may no longer fit, and chewing may be really difficult. Some senile people will no longer use dentures and may take them out and hide them, or just put them in handbag or pockets. If there is a chewing problem, meat should be provided in minced or finely cut-up form. Older people, living alone, may have very poor meals for a variety of reasons. It isn't much fun to cook for one person. If the person is living in a single room, cooking equipment may be pretty sparse. Buying food for one person can be an expensive business.

Some years ago the eating of eggs became a controversial subject. The reason: Eggs contain considerable cholesterol, a substance normally present in many parts of the human body and always present in the blood, where it serves useful purposes. The deposits which form in the blood vessels in atherosclerosis contain a great deal of cholesterol. These deposits hinder the flow of blood and may have something to do with the formation of the clot which causes stoppage in blood flow (this is what happens in the type of heart disease called coronary thrombosis). It was thought that the development of the deposits in the blood vessels would be speeded up if the amount of cholesterol in the blood were raised. For several years it was thought that the concentration of cholesterol in the blood depended on the amount of cholesterol in eaten food. Hence, the eating of eggs was considered to be harmful. The difficulty is that the amount of cholesterol in the blood is influenced only to a very limited extent by the amount of cholesterol in the food. The body can, and does, make cholesterol from starch and sugar, and the amount thus made varies inversely with the cholesterol intake in food. There is no sound reason for not eating eggs unless the individual happens to be one of those rare persons who is allergic to egg protein.

As a matter of fact, eggs are a very desirable food not only because they are palatable but because of what they contain. Eggs are an excellent source of high-quality protein, just as valuable as the protein of meat, fish, or fowl. Eggs contain considerable thiamine, riboflavin, and niacin, and indeed several other vitamins. The iron supplied by eggs is a substantial amount, in comparison with a number of other foods. There are a number of good reasons for eating eggs and there is no sound reason for not eating eggs, except that of allergy. Most people don't need to worry about that. We should have at least three eggs a week, and an egg every day is a good idea. Eggs are easily digested. Eggs make a very good alternative for meat. Eggs are acceptable to most vegetarians.

# CHAPTER | 8

## *Grain Products: Bread, Breakfast Cereals, Corn Meal, Rice*

From an international viewpoint of feeding the world's population, grains and products made from them are the most important foods. They are economical because the yield of human food per acre is much greater than is the case for meat, milk, eggs, and a number of other foods. Those of us who are able to have liberal supplies of meat, milk, eggs, fruits, and vegetables have difficulty in understanding that grain is the main food of a large section of the world's population and that even it may be scarce. Those of us who use wheat foods seldom appreciate that wheat is unobtainable in many areas. Our view is so narrow that we don't see why rice is the main food for about half the population of the world. We even think people who eat rice as the principal food must be queer. We do not realize that rice is eaten in many areas because it is the grain which can be grown in these areas. If we are interested in disposing of surplus storage of wheat, we think that people who have eaten rice for many generations should give up rice and eat our wheat. It never occurs to us that people who we think should eat wheat may not have facilities for milling wheat or for baking bread. We are sure that people who will not help us to get rid of wheat must be queer. Perhaps you have heard, as I have, a statement by a traveling evangelist that we should be Christian and help rice-eating peoples by giving them wheat. It might be more Christian to try to understand the viewpoint and the habits of rice-eating peoples.

In addition to rice and wheat, other grains are used for food. Corn (or maize) can be grown to advantage in some areas and hence it is popular in them. Rye is used by many people in Central Europe. Other grains, like millet, are used in certain districts because they wi' grow under the local conditions.

The grain seeds which are used for food contain thre main parts. On the outside are several layers of bran, hard, outer, protective coating which contains conside able cellulose. This bran coat is likely to contain th amine, other vitamins, iron, phosphorus, and, sometime some calcium. The cellulose in bran gives it laxativ properties, but bran can be irritating in some youn children and in some elderly people. Bran should n be eaten as a laxative unless it is known not to cau irritation in the particular individual. At one end the seed is the young plant or germ. The germ contai an oil which generally has dissolved in it, appreciabl amounts of vitamin E (of value to some species of animals but of doubtful value for humans) and carotene.

The germ is likely, also, to be a good source of thiamine, other vitamins, iron, and phosphorus. The main part of the seed, called the endosperm, contains starch and protein, designed by nature to nourish the young plant as it grows. The protein is not high-quality protein and generally lacks one or more of the essential amino acids. In the germ there is a smaller amount of better quality protein.

When grains are prepared for human food, the bran and germ are commonly removed, no matter which grain is used. The endosperm, eaten by humans, is a very economical source of starch and incomplete protein, but it is not a good source of vitamins, or of nutrients like iron and phosphorus. In 1918 a committee of the Royal Society of Britain reported that, if ninety per cent of wheat were used by humans in place of eighty per cent, people would receive thirty-four pounds of additional protein and nearly three hundred thousand additional calories from each ton of wheat. The committee did not include the additional quantities of vitamins, of iron, and of other nutrients. The use of an increased proportion of wheat would result in dark flour, which is not popular.

While greater nutritive value and more economy would result from the eating of the whole grain, there are some practical points to consider. Whole grains and whole grain products (whole wheat flour, for example) do not keep as well during storage as do refined products (such as white flour). Whole grain products are not digested as thoroughly as refined products, and the contained bran may be an irritant in the intestines of some people. We should face the fact, also, that a great many people do not like and will not eat whole grain foods;

this is as true of rice as it is of wheat. Those of us who have liberal intakes of meat, milk, and eggs, do not need to be concerned about the nutritive value of bread. In areas in which grain is the main food, the nutritive value of the grain product eaten is of great importance.

It is of advantage to consider briefly the nutritive value and the usefulness of various grains and of foods made from them.

### Wheat

Most of the people in the United States, in Canada, in Britain, and in several European countries regard wheat as *the* food grain. Bread, made from wheat flour, has been in use for many centuries, and it has been labeled the staff of life. In recent years, the consumption of bread has decreased; it is not as important a food as it used to be.

There are various kinds of wheat and the composition is not entirely uniform. On the average wheat contains about seventy-five per cent starch, about twelve per cent protein, and about two per cent oil or fat. Hard wheats contain somewhat more protein than soft wheats and are more useful for bread-making. Durum wheat has more protein than either hard or soft wheat and is used for the production of macaroni and spaghetti.

The grains of wheat contain the three main parts described above and the distribution of nutrients in the bran, germ, and endosperm have been noted. To produce flour, wheat kernels are ground and the ground material sieved. Authentic whole wheat or graham flour contains the entire kernels and hence the full nutritive value of the kernels. Whole wheat flour is brown, has a characteristic flavor. White flour (to produce white bread) became fashionable in the nineteeth century and white bread became the acceptable kind. The bran and germ are removed in the production of white flour and, with them, a considerable portion of the nutritive value of whole wheat. In recent years, factory-made vitamins have become available at such low cost that three vitamins can be added to white flour to counterbalance some of the losses brought about in milling flour. Flour with added vitamins is called "enriched." A more accurate name would be "partially restored," since not all milling losses are made good. Over a period of some years there was considerable excitement about the nutritive value of white bread. People were urged to use whole wheat bread. Enthusiasts still exist who claim that some human ills are caused by eating white bread instead of whole wheat. Admittedly, the nutritive value of authentic whole wheat bread is greater than that of white bread, even when enriched flour is used. The consumption of bread has declined; it is now used to a fairly small extent by many people. These people are eating generous quantities of meat and eggs. To them the nutritive value of bread is of slight importance.

Bread is an economical source of starch and hence of energy. The protein in bread is obtained cheaply in comparison with protein from meat and eggs. True, the bread protein is not complete and does lack some essential amino acids. The incompleteness can be taken care of by eating proteins which supply the missing amino acids. Proteins from meat, milk, and eggs have this effect. Bread-and-milk is a good food.

In modern society bread has one very real advantage; it can be used to make sandwiches. A lot can be said in praise of a good ham sandwich or a good cheese sandwich. In one fell swoop we obtain an economical source of energy and a good source of protein, if a decent amount of ham or cheese has been put into the sandwich.

As a consequence of economic prosperity and also because of an increasing emphasis on getting weight down, bread has become an unfashionable food for many persons in the United States and Canada. We have money available to buy extravagant cars and extravagant foods. No wonder people in the underdeveloped countries envy us. There is still a good argument for bread and a sensible bit of advice is to eat four or more slices of bread a day, unless we are engaged in rapid weight reduction.

Of course, wheat is used in foods other than bread. Some of these with flour as a major ingredient are pretty well akin to bread. Personally, I like hot biscuits, especially homemade ones. Perhaps you are familiar with cooking in the Southern states and know all about the kind of hot biscuits I mean.

Macaroni, spagetti, vermicelli, and noodles are made from durum wheat which has the high content of protein necessary to give body to these foods. These foods are economical and can be made not only tasty but nutritious by adding generous quantities of cheese and meat. I favor a mixture of macaroni, milk and a lot of cheese. That mixture is a cheap source of many nutrients. In addition it has a grand flavor. I do not own stock in any macaroni company or in any dairy or cheese company but I do like good food, especially when it is also economical.

### Corn

The use of corn for human food has been both damned and praised. This grain is called maize in Britain, in which country corn is a name for wheat. Corn is a very important crop in the United States but not for direct use as food for humans. The main use of corn is to feed to farm animals. Most of the corn raised in the United States is turned into beef, pork, eggs, and milk.

Like other grains, a kernel of corn consists of three main parts. The outer layer is removed, not by milling as in the case of wheat, but by soaking. The germ of corn contains about thirty per cent oil which is separated and sold as corn oil. Corn endosperm has about the same proportion of protein as does wheat endosperm. Corn protein is more incomplete than wheat protein.

When whole corn is softened by steaming, the hulls removed, and the germ loosened in a hulling machine, the horny, starchy part of the kernel is left in coarse pieces. This is called "hominy." Hominy is ground to make "grits." Hominy and grits are popular foods in the Southern states. Corn meal can be made by grinding the entire kernel to give old-style corn meal, or by grinding the endosperm to make new-style corn meal. Corn meal can be used to make a number of very appetizing foods (corn bread, spoon bread, corn-meal mush or porridge, to name a few common ones).

Corn has been praised because it is an economical food with a characteristic and very popular flavor. The use of corn as a "vegetable" should not be overlooked. Corn-on-the-cob is a very pleasant food, at least for people in North America. Canned corn and frozen corn are useful "vegetables." In many areas corn is a prolific crop providing an economical food. The Mexican tortilla, made from corn, is the bread of many families in that country.

Corn has been damned because of its relation to

pellagra. Its prevalence was so often associated with reliance on corn as the main food that pellagra was labeled the "corn-eater's disease." Pellagra is caused by a lack of the vitamin, niacin. This vitamin is supplied by meat, eggs, and some other foods. The corn-eaters who developed pellagra had small intakes of foods which are excellent sources of niacin. The body can obtain niacin pre-formed in certain foods and in another, indirect way. One of the amino acids, tryptophane, can be turned into niacin in the body. Corn contains very little niacin and little or no tryptophane. The people who got pellagra did so because their meals lacked both niacin and its precursor, tryptophane. The deficiencies of corn are of minor importance if meat and eggs are available and are eaten. Pellagra disappeared from the Southern states because improvement in economic conditions made possible the more generous use of meat and other foods which supply both niacin and tryptophane.

## Rye

This grain is hardier than wheat and can be grown in Northern Europe where wheat cannot be raised. The food value of rye is very similar to that of wheat. Rye bread is, of course, a staple food in countries in which rye is grown as the principal grain and rye bread has become very popular in the United States and in Canada in recent years, especially with salami or with cheese. There is no sound reason for urging people who are accustomed to rye bread to replace it with wheat bread.

## Rice

To most North Americans rice is a food to be used occasionally in place of potatoes or as a dessert, particularly in institutions and in boardinghouses. For half of the population of the world, rice is the main food.

Rice kernels have an outside husk which is removed before rice is used as food. Inside the husk but on the outside of the kernel is a brown layer of bran. If this is left on, rice is called "brown rice." Removal of this layer of bran gives white or "polished" rice, the kind that most of us are familiar with. The bran layer contains a good deal of the vitamin, thiamine; the endosperm (polished rice) has a very low content of thiamine. When people live on polished rice as the main food and foods containing thiamine are scarce, they develop a deficiency of thiamine. The resultant disease is beriberi. Brown rice has a distinctive flavor, not liked by people who have been accustomed to polished rice. Moreover, brown rice deteriorates more quickly in storage. Thiamine can be added to white rice and trials of such treated rice have shown that its use can prevent beriberi.

### Breakfast Cereals

Scottish people reading the previous part of the chapter may have decided that some mention should have been made of oats. This grain is used mainly as a breakfast cereal and this food has many virtues. Oatmeal or oat flakes have a good content of thiamine, of iron, and of several other nutrients. Oatmeal porridge is a healthful, tasty, and economical food.

A wide variety of breakfast cereals is available. Many different prepared ones can be purchased, with or without space-ships or other premiums. They are not identical in nutritive value or in cost. Breakfast cereals can be divided into two main groups: (1) Those with the nutritive value of whole grains, such as oatmeal or oat flakes, wheat flakes, shredded wheat; (2) those having less nutritive value than whole grains. A good example is corn flakes. Corn flakes are made by rolling thin the softened endosperm of corn and toasting the thin flakes. Many of the prepared cereals in the United States have added vitamins.

Prepared cereals are likely to be much more expensive than those which are bought in bulk and cooked. Oatmeal and wheat flakes are good sources of thiamine and of iron, and they are cheap.

Bran breakfast foods are often used to combat constipation. The safe thing to do is to see your doctor to find the cause of the constipation. Bran may be irritating to the intestinal tract of young children and of elderly people and should be used with care.

Other cereals may be used for breakfast. I realize that corn-meal mush does not have as much nutritive value as oatmeal but I like it occasionally for variety. By the way, variety is a good idea even in breakfast. We don't need to have the same food every morning.

Breakfast cereals provide intriguing examples of silly advertising. A sedentary person, like a professor, cannot be turned into a champion athlete, or any kind of an athlete, by eating a particular cereal. Recently, people have been urged to eat a special cereal to obtain protein. One ounce of the cereal in question (an average serving) contains about as much protein as four ounces of milk. The milk is cheaper and the protein in it is complete; the protein in the cereal is incomplete. Pops and crackles may be entertaining but they do not add to the health value of breakfast. The old motto, Let the buyer beware, is useful to remember when shopping for breakfast cereals.

# CHAPTER 9

# Sweet Foods: Nice to Eat, but—

People in the United States and in Canada eat about one quarter of a pound of sugar per day. Sugar is a cheap food but it is not eaten primarily as a food. It provides the most universally used flavor. Whether it is a flavor or not, the average per capita consumption of sugar provides about five hundred calories a day—and nothing else. Refined sugar is purified carbohydrate. It is a source of energy and as such is useful. But sugar has no other real nutritive value. Energy can be obtained from a variety of foods and many of these will supply protein, vitamins and various nutrient elements.

Ordinarily, we do not eat sugar by itself. We don't take a spoonful of sugar and eat it. Sugar is put into tea or coffee, it is used to sweeten candy and ice cream, and it is added, again for sweetening purposes, to cake, pie, a variety of desserts, and also to or with breakfast cereals. It is a main ingredient in soft drinks.

Sweet foods have an advantage which has been recognized for many years. They give a feeling of satisfaction. This is the reason for ending a meal with a sweet dessert. Sweet foods contribute sugar to the blood quickly and the increase in the amount of sugar in the blood lessens or stops hunger. This effect can be of value to people who are on reducing diets. Meals in reducing diets may be pretty meager. A dessert with some sugar and yet not too high in calories can provide some satisfaction. However, the satisfaction value of sweet foods can be unfortunate, particularly in the case of children. If sweet foods are eaten shortly before a meal, hunger for the meal can be reduced so much that a decent meal will not be eaten. This is the reason why it is unwise to give sweet food to children in the hour before a meal. It might be better to say it is *one* reason, since there is another.

There is a great concern about the terrific amount of tooth decay. The reasons for the prevalence of tooth decay are not completely clear but there is a good deal of sound information which should be known to parents and to children. Tooth decay is caused by an attack on tooth enamel by acid. The acid is produced by bacteria living in the mouth. The bacteria produce the acid from starch and sugar used for food by the bacteria. If starch and sugar are close to the surface of the tooth, the acid which the bacteria produce is handily located to attack and dissolve the structure of the tooth.

A number of things can be done to prevent the formation of the acid or to lessen its effect. If we could prevent bacteria from living in the mouth, the problem of tooth decay would disappear, but there is no good method for doing that. It is obvious that keeping starch and sugar from sticking to teeth or remaining between the teeth would help greatly. It is hence obvious that the teeth should be cleaned and the mouth rinsed shortly after eating. This practice should be taught to children at an early age and should be encouraged so that it becomes a persistent habit. Another very useful procedure for helping to prevent tooth decay is to reduce the amount of sugar-containing foods given to children. During the Second World War sugar was scarce in Britain and in most European countries and sugar was rationed so severely that its consumption was greatly reduced. In those countries tooth decay was sharply decreased. There is a large amount of evidence that a reduction in the use of sweet foods by children helps to lessen tooth decay. It has been said that children must have a need for sugar in their bodies because they crave it. They are not born with that craving; it is created by unwise feeding. Sticky candy is particularly bad because it adheres to the teeth. Drinking milk gives children calcium for the formation of bones and teeth. The milk does not have to be flavored with chocolate and sugar. Breakfast cereal does not need to be flavored with sugar.

Tooth decay can be decreased in another obvious way by bringing about the formation of teeth which are harder and more resistant to the attack by acids. Four nutrients are needed for the formation of teeth: calcium, phosphorus, vitamin D, and ascorbic acid. The formation of teeth starts before the baby is born. Children will have stronger and better formed teeth if supplies of these nutrients are available to the mother in the four months before the baby is born and to children until all the second teeth have erupted. These nutrients are not provided by cake, pastry, candy, and soft drinks. Calcium is furnished by milk, phosphorus by milk and a number of other foods, ascorbic acid by fruits and vegetables (especially citrus fruit).

In recent years it has been proved that harder and more resistant teeth are formed if a small amount of fluorine is available during the period of tooth formation. In a few districts there is sufficient fluorine in the soil to contribute fluorine to water in an amount adequate for the formation of resistant teeth. In such areas there is much less tooth decay. Fluorine can be added to community water supplies. Tests of the procedure have shown that a very marked reduction in tooth decay is the result. The fluoridation of water supplies has been opposed and one of the arguments is that fluorine is poisonous. Sodium fluoride (a compound used to raise the fluorine content of water) is called "rat poison." It is true that sodium fluoride can be used to kill rats and other pests. In the amount used in fluoridated water, sodium fluoride is harmless; it is even beneficial. A large dose of caffeine (the stimulant in tea and coffee) will cause death but a great number of people drink tea and coffee. Many other examples could be given of substances which are harmless in small amounts and lethal in large amounts. The possible harmful effects of adding fluorine to water in proportions which reduce tooth decay have been very thoroughly investigated in several countries. These studies have proved that fluoridation of water is harmless and that it is beneficial. There is only one catch to the fluoridation of water supplies. What about farm children? A safe method for supplying fluorine to children living in areas not having community water supplies is needed.

Parents who wish their children to have strong, healthy

teeth protected against decay should do these things.

1. See that mother has good intakes of calcium, phosphorus, vitamin D and ascorbic acid during the second half of pregnancy. Such intakes can be assured by the mother taking 1½ pints of milk a day, citrus fruit or juice once a day, 400 units of vitamin D a day.
2. Do not encourage children to want sweet foods. The use of cake, pie, candy and soft drinks should not be encouraged but should be discouraged.
3. Help children to develop the habit of cleaning teeth after meals and of rinsing the mouth if cleaning is not possible.
4. Support the fluoridation of water supplies.

Tooth decay is far too prevalent. We can all help to prevent it.

There is another aspect to the use of sweet foods. It is true that they do furnish energy, that sugar is cheap, that sweet foods at the end of a meal give a feeling of satisfaction. It is true, also, that sweet foods are not good buys from the viewpoint of meeting needs for various nutrients. Milk, cheese, fruits, vegetables, eggs, are much better buys in the long run. When there is need to economize in food purchases, it is sensible to get the most value possible. Cake, pastry, candy, soft drinks, are not economical. Buying them wastes money which could be better spent.

A rather prevalent illusion about many soft drinks is that they do not contain much sugar and are low in calories. Teen-age girls will refuse to drink milk but will use soft drinks. There are soft drinks which are low in calories. However, many soft drinks contain more sugar than might be suspected. A serving of eight ounces of a popular drink contains one ounce of sugar and has a calorie value of 100. This is the same number of calories provided by eight ounces of orange juice, which is an excellent source of ascorbic acid and other essential nutrients not present in the soft drink. It should be noted that eight ounces of skim milk, containing calcium, riboflavin, and high-quality protein, has a calorie value of 87. If you want to think about the costs of foods, try comparing the cost of skim milk, orange juice, and a popular soft drink. In the city in which this is written and at the time of writing, skim milk delivered to the house in quart bottles is one-half the cost per ounce of the soft drink in question bought in a carton of six eight-ounce bottles (if the bottles are returned and the deposit collected). It's a good plan to get your money's worth in buying foods.

If you are concerned with losing weight and in staying slim, you had better know the calorie value of some commonly used sweet foods, especially when the small contributions of other nutrient values is remembered. Here are the energy values of some frequently eaten sweet foods:

1 piece of chocolate layer cake .......... 410 calories
(1/10 of a cake, ten-inch diameter)
1 piece of lemon meringue pie .......... 302 calories
(1/7 of a nine-inch pie)
1 ounce caramels .................... 118 calories

These few calorie values carry a moral: These foods, and others like them, must be avoided if you are concerned with losing weight or if you are anxious to stay slim. Sweets are a cause of obesity.

In recent years spurious claims have been made for several sweet foods. Blackstrap or crude, dark molasses has been claimed to prevent or cure arthritis and a variety of other diseases. The molasses story seems to have been started by a pianist, and pamphlets, said to have been written by this pianist, were circulated from stores selling "health foods." There should be question marks after both "health" and "foods"—those shops are made possible by gullibility and ignorance. The molasses story was widely touted by Gayelord Hauser. Crude molasses contains sugar, some iron and some of the B vitamins. So do many other foods. Crude molasses has *no* special virtue. At the peak of the craze for molasses, a drug firm seeking to sell molasses without committing fraud, put out bottles of molasses labeled: "This molasses is good for any condition for which molasses is beneficial." There's a really truthful claim.

The expression, "quick energy," is used frequently in advertisements for certain syrups and breakfast cereals. The meaning is doubtful but the impression is given that the use of these foods will give people a lift in a few minutes. Solutions of sugar are quickly digested and absorbed, but whether that will produce suddenly a feeling of elation and a capacity for doing work or exercise is not so clear. This expression is a kind of half-truth intended to give a false impression of the value of a specific product.

Despite the prevalence of the "sweet tooth" possessed by many people, and despite the feeling of satisfaction provided by sweet foods, we could save money, teeth, and health by cutting down on sweet foods and using foods which give better value. Fruit is satisfactory for dessert and is preferable to a food which supplies only starch and sugar, as is the case with puddings.

# CHAPTER 10

# Good Meals for Health, Pleasure,
## and Economy

Many people have the notion that the selection of foods to meet health needs makes meals unpalatable and that eating for health is a kind of penance. That notion is so false that it needs to be dispelled. Meals should be enjoyed. They should be pleasant interludes in life. What sort of meals should we have?

In Chapter 3 the needs of the body were discussed and in six subsequent chapters various kinds of foods were described in relation to meeting needs. Let's summarize those needs:

1. We need food to supply energy to keep the body warm, to enable life to continue, to give growth.
2. We need protein for growth and to maintain the body.

3. We need calcium, phosphorus, vitamin D, and ascorbic acid for the development of healthy teeth and bones. Calcium, phosphorus, and ascorbic acid are needed throughout life. Adults, except pregnant women, do not need vitamin D.

4. We need iron to maintain the blood in a healthy state. Don't worry about "tired" blood—whatever that is. We need iodine for the work of the thyroid gland.

5. We need a number of vitamins for normal functions in the body.

All of these needs, except for vitamin D, can be satisfied by eating commonly available foods. To meet these needs, we should use the following foods:

*Milk:* At least one half pint a day for adults.
   At least one pint a day for children (up to 10-12 years).
   At least 1½ pints a day for teen-agers, for expectant and nursing mothers.
   Milk contains high-quality protein, calcium and riboflavin.

*Fruit:* At least one serving of fruit a day *plus* one serving of oranges, grapefruit, orange juice, or grapefruit juice.
   Fruit, particularly citrus fruit, is used to supply ascorbic acid.

*Vegetables:* At least one serving of potatoes a day *and* two servings of other vegetables a day.
   Vegetables supply ascorbic acid, iron, vitamin A, and other nutrients. Green-leaf and yellow vegetables are cheap sources of vitamin A.

*Meat, Fish, Fowl:* At least one serving of meat, or fish,

or fowl a day. These foods give high-quality protein, thiamine, niacin, iron.

*Bread and Cereals:* Four slices of bread a day—or more,
*if needed.*

One serving of breakfast cereal having whole-
grain value. Bread and breakfast cereals are
cheap sources of energy, of thiamine, riboflavin,
niacin and, in some cases, iron.

*Eggs:* At least 3 eggs a week, because eggs contain high-
quality protein, iron, thiamine, riboflavin, and
niacin.

*Cheese:* At least 3 servings (an ounce or more) a week
since cheese is a cheap source of high-quality protein and of calcium.

*Vitamin D:* Children, teen-agers, expectant mothers (in
the second half of pregnancy) should have 400
units a day. More than that amount is *not* needed.
Vitamin D is added to evaporated milk and can
be obtained from drug preparations.

The quantities of foods specified above are for
normal persons of "ideal" or less than ideal
weight. The total quantities, as advised for
adults, will give 1700-1800 calories a day. If you
need a greater supply of calories you can use
larger servings.

Three meals a day has been the custom for most people for many years. These meals may be breakfast, lunch,
and dinner, or breakfast, dinner, and supper, depending
on which arrangement is convenient. Social prestige
frequently enters into the matter and some people think
it is more elegant to have dinner in the evening. Changes
in the character of meals have occurred in recent years
and some of the changes are undesirable. Forty years
ago meals were family affairs and they could be eaten

leisurely. In recent years this pattern has been altered, at least in cities and suburbs, to gobbling hurriedly prepared food placed on counters or built-in little tables. May the saints deliver us from "eating areas." Cooking is no longer a fine art, to be cherished and passed on to daughters. What is the use of bothering about cooking? Anyway, we just have to heat up prepared and packaged foods which have no distinctive flavor so they must be covered with catsup (or ketchup, if you prefer). A lot of people seem to have lost their sense of taste.

I am in favor of home-cooked meals, nicely served, eaten leisurely with conversation with the family around the table. This is awfully old-fashioned, isn't it? It can be done if there is any interest in a good life.

The prevalent meal pattern is little or no breakfast, a light lunch, and a heavy dinner. Most people would feel better, physically and mentally, if the total amount were divided more evenly and if meals were pleasant and more leisurely. We hurry like mad to get somewhere— what do we do when we get there?

Breakfast is the meal most often neglected. After being without food for eight hours or more, we need a decent breakfast. It is worth while to get up fifteen to twenty minutes earlier and have breakfast. Why leave home in such a frightful rush? It's a great advantage to health and to peace of mind to get up a bit earlier, dress more slowly, eat a good breakfast with the family. Choose the nearest exit—walk—*do not run* is good advice at home too. Those of us who read the comics are accustomed to Blondie handing Dagwood a cup of coffee in the hall—poor Dagwood.

Here is my idea of a good breakfast:

An orange, or half a grapefruit, or at least 4 ounces
of orange or grapefruit juice.
A healthy serving of porridge (oatmeal or wheat
flake) with a lot of milk.
A poached egg on toast.
A cup of *good* coffee.

A food rich in protein is advisable with breakfast.
Such foods as eggs, meat, fish, or cheese are useful protein
sources. Cheese for breakfast is better than you think, if
you haven't tried it. You may like fish for breakfast—so
do I, but not every morning. We don't need to have the
same foods every morning. Variety for breakfast is a good
plan. Citrus fruit or juice at the start is pleasant and it
does whet the appetite.

One of the undesirable features of European travel is
the so-called Continental breakfast. For one thing it
isn't enough food for a morning of moving around and
where does the coffee come from? Coffee as served in
most hotels in Paris seems to have been made the night
before, grounds from several days mixed in, and the
mixture heated. French people may be good cooks but
what about breakfast coffee?

I realize that the preparation of a good breakfast takes
time. Well, it's worth it. If breakfast has been nicely
prepared, it should be savored. That can't be done standing up. Let's start the day peacefully and in comfort.
Dividends will be evident all morning.

City life is a mess in many ways. Grabbing a bit of
lunch, with catsup on it, at a lunch counter is a sorry
business. Is it really necessary? One of the advantages
of living on a farm or in a small town is that it is possible
to go home and have a nice meal at noon. The noon

meal should be more than a hamburg on a bun or a malted milk, or even just a cup of coffee.

The make-up of the main meal (dinner) eaten at noon will be considered presently. If the noon meal is lunch, what should it be like? If lunch is brought from home it is likely to contain sandwiches. They should have a protein-rich filling such as cheese, meat, or eggs. A carbo-hydrate filling like jelly with bread is not a good com-bination. With the sandwiches a jar of vegetable salad is a help. Fruit, with or without cookies, is a good dessert. The beverage should be milk, or, in cold weather, cocoa made with milk and no water. If lunch is bought it can include meat or fish or fowl, but they should not be re-garded as essential. A bowl of hearty vegetable soup, a sandwich with a cheese or meat filling, fruit and milk is a good lunch but not too substantial. Lunch should include a good source of protein and that source need not be meat. In cold weather one hot dish is pleasant and the hot dish could be macaroni and cheese (plenty of cheese) or even baked beans. Milk should be the beverage for lunch. If you are interested in weight loss, a salad, vegetable with some meat, or fruit is useful. Lunch can be nourishing, pleasant and restful. Taking just a bit longer for lunch instead of gulping it can make lunch a rest before the afternoon.

Dinner, whether at noon or in the evening, is likely to be a substantial meal. It's really better to spread food a little more evenly through the day. If a man comes home tired and worried, it's a good idea to relax for a while before dinner. One method of promoting relaxa-tion is to sit down in a comfortable chair and sip a glass of sherry or a *moderate* amount of alcohol in some other form. This lowers the blood pressure, gives a feeling of comfort, and stimulates the feeling of hunger.

The mainstay of dinner is likely to be meat, fish, or fowl with vegetables. Dinner can be started with soup; if made with meat stock, soup may promote hunger. Desserts of wide varieties can be used. Extra milk can be introduced in custard or in ice cream. Fruit makes a good dessert, particularly if the person is concerned about weight. Tea or coffee may be the beverage, but for children it should be milk. Of course, it would be an advantage for children and for adults if the whole family drank milk.

These recommended meal patterns are not strange and they can be appetizing and pleasant. Some of you may regard a substantial breakfast as either unobtainable or unsuitable. Try it for a while and you are likely to continue.

It is cheaper to have healthy meals than it is to purchase nonessential foods which waste money. Many families spend considerable money in buying cake, pie, candy, and soft drinks. These foods furnish energy but do not contribute appreciable protein, vitamins or other nutrients. The foods recommended above are essential because they satisfy our nutrition requirements; they give good value for the money spent on them.

√    A wise housewife plans meals several days or a week ahead to ensure that they are attractive and healthful. Such planning saves time and money in shopping and in meal preparation. When shopping, it should be remembered that foods in bulk packages are usually cheaper than those in small, fancy packages. The most expensive grades of canned foods are not likely to have any more nutrition value than cheaper grades. Cheaper cuts of meat are as nutritious as more expensive ones and can be made just as palatable by proper cooking. Foods in season are a good buy because they are at their cheapest price and possess their greatest food value. Leftovers can be made into appetizing dishes. Wise planning and economical marketing aid in having good meals.

Meals can be made more interesting by using a greater variety of foods and even more variety in methods of cooking, as we have suggested earlier. It's a good idea not to have a particular dish on the same day each week. Monday should not be a stew day or meatloaf day. A wide variety of meats and meat products is available. One kind of food likely to be too much restricted is vegetables. Meals can be more interesting if a wide variety of vegetables is used. If the family rebels about a new vegetable, don't give up. Not only does variety make meals—and life—more interesting, variety increases the likelihood of getting needed nutrients.

The palatability of meals depends largely on cooking. Cooking *is* an art and good cooking should be encouraged before it is forced off the scene by living in a hurry with factory-prepared, ready-to-serve foods and meals.

The main reason for cookery is to make food digestible, palatable, and attractive. Moderately cooked meat is more digestible than either raw meat or overcooked meat. Cooked starch is more digestible than raw starch. Cooking can cause a reduction in nutritive value. Some nutrients are destroyed by oxidation and this process is accelerated by heat. Nutrients which are soluble in water can be extracted from foods when they are cooked in water.

Losses in nutritive value caused by cooking can be re-

duced. Sometimes it is necessary to work out a compromise. Meat cooked slowly at low temperature is more
tender and generally more tasty; however, the prolonged
exposure to heat increases destruction of thiamine, riboflavin, and niacin. It is probably better to guard the
palatability and tenderness of the meat.

In the case of vegetable cookery, no compromise is
needed. Measures which help to conserve nutritive value
also conserve appearance, taste, and general attractive-
ness. There is nothing worse than overcooked, drowned,
brown cabbage. When vegetables are cooked in water,
the smallest possible quantity of water should be used,
vegetables should be left in fairly large pieces, and cooking continued only until the vegetable is tender enough
to eat. Cooked vegetables should be served and eaten
as soon as possible after they are cooked. Water should
be boiling before vegetables are placed in it and the
utensil should be covered. The steam-cooking of vegetables is better than cooking in water, so far as nutritive
value is concerned. If you are interested in a different
method of cooking cabbage, try cooking it in fat or oil.
A thin layer of oil or fat on the bottom of a saucepan
with the cabbage resting on it will do the trick.

Foods can be selected for health and for pleasure at
the same time. Meals can and should be attractive. Good
cooking is of prime importance. The notion that meals
will be unpleasant if we select foods to meet nutrition
needs is ridiculous nonsense. The attractive meals which
can be prepared from a variety of good foods will make
life more pleasant, more interesting, and more healthful.
It may be necessary to give up some silly notions and to
change food habits a bit. The changes will be worth
while.

# CHAPTER 11

# *Good Meals for Betty and Tommy*

Betty and Tommy are nice children. You probably know that there are two kinds of children; our own little angels and the neighbors' little devils. We want Betty and Tommy to grow up normally, to be healthy, fond of exercise, and top-grade mentally. Of course, we also want them, Betty especially, to be good-looking.

Let's hope that they got off to a good start. If mother ate sensibly during the last four months before the babies were born, the babies were healthier at birth. We do hope that Betty and Tommy were breast-fed, for six months, anyway. Breast milk is the best and the safest food for babies. Incidentally, a mother who is breast-feeding her baby needs extra calcium and extra protein for the production of milk; both nutrients can be obtained by drinking at least 1½ pints of milk a day in addition to good meals.

Even in breast-fed babies, and always in babies who are

not breast-fed, two nutrient deficiencies need to be guarded against. Babies need protection against scurvy and rickets. The first disease is prevented by a supply of ascorbic acid, obtained in orange juice. Rickets is prevented by a supply of 400 units a day of vitamin D. Concentrated preparations of vitamin D are available; a few drops of a concentrated preparation placed directly into the baby's mouth will do. The giving of both orange juice and vitamin D should be started when the baby is two weeks old.

At three months of age most babies are ready for cereal in addition to milk feedings. Usually one of the many brands of precooked, infant cereal is used because of convenience. The cereal is mixed with cooked, boiled milk, feeding formula, or water to make a thin gruel. As the baby becomes older the cereal feeding can be made thicker and a greater amount fed.

Milk, even breast milk, contains very little iron. When born, the baby generally contains a store of iron, sufficient for several months. By the age of five months, food sources of iron are advisable and it is now common practice to give babies a variety of puréed vegetables, eggs, and finely chopped meat. These foods supply iron and other essential nutrients. Their use provides, also, an introduction to a variety of foods needed for growth and needed throughout life.

By nine months of age most babies have adapted themselves to three meals a day and within a few months will be attempting to feed themselves. In the second year the rate of growth is much less than in the first year and food needs are consequently reduced. Parents may not realize this change in growth rate and in food needs. They become disturbed about the unwillingness of the child to eat as much as they think is necessary. For this reason, feeding problems, created by parents, start to develop. Attempts to force the child to eat more food than needed leads to trouble. In this second year it is an advantage to have children eat by themselves to avoid distractions and to help them to give attention only to eating.

Suitable meals for children during the second year are ones like these:

*Breakfast:* small portion of cereal with milk
           egg or crisp bacon
           toast
           a cup of whole or skim milk.
*Mid-morning:* orange juice
           vitamin D (400 units)
           plain biscuit, if the youngster is hungry.
*Noon meal:* chopped meat
           small serving of baked or mashed potato
           small serving of chopped vegetable
           toast or bread
           milk pudding, custard or fruit
           1 cup of milk
*Mid-afternoon:* a banana or a plain biscuit
*Evening meal:* cereal, or egg, or cottage cheese
           chopped vegetable
           fruit or milk pudding
           1 cup milk

During the second year children should not be given ice cream, candy, soft drinks, nuts, popcorn, cucumbers, corn, pastry, pickles, spices, or seasonings.

Between the end of the second year and by the time the child has started to school, parents should foster and encourage by example and by tact the formation of good food habits. Some food habits can be called not only desirable but essential for healthy growth. The daily drinking of milk and the development of a regard for milk as *the* beverage is an essential habit. Children are unlikely to want milk if father thinks of milk as food for babies. A highly desirable outlook toward food is a willingness to try new foods and to eat a variety. It is useful to encourage children to like the natural flavors of foods: cereal without sugar—milk without sugar and chocolate —eggs without catsup.

A question which is asked very frequently is, How do you get children to eat the foods they should eat? Not by nagging, is one answer. Putting the eating of a particular food on a basis of "it's good for you" will not only not help, but may keep the children from eating the food in question. Making food the basis of either punishment or reward is inadvisable. This is true particularly of sweet foods. The giving of candy as a reward for good behavior is a simple method of developing a sweet tooth. Badgering a youngster about the use of food gives the youngster a weapon to wield against parents. The child soon realizes that he can agree to eat something if a concession is provided in return. It is easy to see where this leads. Whether a child develops good habits depends on the attitude of the parents. To start with, we provide for children foods which are selected on a health basis. We set an example by eating those foods ourselves. We give the child the impression that he is expected to eat those foods and we are surprised if he doesn't. Sometimes, older relatives can spoil the situation by telling about what they ate when they were young—which may be quite different from modern methods of feeding children. It is never wise to make an issue of a child's refusal to eat. Good food habits should be a matter of course.

As children become older they should be given information about the reasons for sensible food selection. All too frequently this has to be done in school because many parents don't know or don't care. An understanding of bodily needs and how those needs are met is essential to ensure suitable choice of foods.

Children should have a good breakfast before they go to school. The breakfast should be more than a hurried snack and it should include citrus fruit, or juice, cereal having whole grain value with plenty of milk, a good source of protein (such as an egg), bread or toast and milk. While it is essential for children to have a suitable amount of milk, too much milk may keep youngsters from eating other needed foods. Children under eight who are fond of milk can drink too much at the start of a meal. It's a good plan to give not more than half a cup of milk with a meal and then let children have additional milk after the meal is eaten.

It is now common practice in most areas to provide noon meals in schools. However, if lunch is taken from home, real thought should be given to its make-up. Lunch, carried or secured in school, should be attractive, appetizing, and should contain foods needed for healthy growth. The mainstay of lunch from home may be sandwiches. The filling should be an excellent source of high-quality protein, such as meat, fish, poultry, eggs, or cheese. Peanut butter is fairly satisfactory; jelly is not. Variety in sandwich fillings makes lunch more interesting. Raw vegetables in salad in a jar, or in segments, have several advantages. They provide ascorbic acid, iron and other essential nutrients, and they encourage chewing. Fruit is much better than cake or pie. The beverage should be milk, or in cold weather cocoa made with milk.

Parents should be concerned about school meals. Menus should be based on the selection of foods to meet the needs of health. Candy, gum, and soft drinks should not be on sale in school cafeterias or lunchrooms. Kitchens should be clean, food should be properly prepared and properly cooked. If nutrition is included in health education in the school, the school meals should be the practical demonstration of classroom teaching. Children cannot be expected to drink milk in a school cafeteria if the teachers, after urging milk in the classroom, drink coffee at noon in sight of the children.

Adolescents generally need considerable food, and boys especially eat amounts which seem to be terrific. About the time of puberty there is a spurt in growth and this increases food needs. The real needs will not be met unless they are understood and unless foods are selected to meet the needs. Increases in height and weight are accompanied by increases in the length and thickness of bones. Consequently, there is an increased need for calcium—best obtained from milk and cheese. If Tommy, now fifteen, drinks a quart of milk a day, don't be alarmed. He needs at least 1½ pints of milk a day to supply calcium. If Betty is fourteen, she has an increased need for calcium, too. Unfortunately, she may not drink milk because she thinks milk is fattening and she is anxious to stay slim. Milk is less fattening than cake or pie, and is a needed food.

Betty's interest in keeping slim is understandable; she wants to be attractive. This desire to stay slim can be satisfied and, indeed, encouraged. The prevention of overweight and obesity is much easier than the cure. The main point to emphasize with Betty is that food can be selected to meet essential needs for protein, for vitamins, for calcium, and other nutrients and still not be excessive in calories. A number of suggestions can be made to Betty to help her keep slim and healthy. There are foods which she needs to complete growth, for maintenance, and to meet health needs. These foods should be regarded by Betty as essential:

*Milk:* 1½ pints a day of skim milk—calorie value, 280

*Citrus fruit:* 1 medium orange, or ½ grapefruit, or 4 ounces of orange or grapefruit juice—calorie value, 60-70

*Other fruit:* 1 serving a day—calorie value, 50-80

*Vegetables:* 1 small serving potatoes a day—calorie value, 100

2 servings other vegetables a day—calorie value, 70-80

*Meat, Fish, or Fowl:* 1 serving a day—calorie value, 300

*Breakfast Cereal* (whole grain type):   1 serving a day—calorie value, 150

*Bread:* 3 slices a day with butter or margarine—calorie value, 300

These foods are essential for Betty because they can be used to give three attractive meals a day, and because they contain protein, vitamins, calcium, iron and other nutrients. The total calorie yield from these essential foods will not exceed 1,400 a day. This will not be enough for Betty's needs and would constitute a reducing diet, bringing about a weight loss. Therefore, two other foods should be included. Betty should have at least three eggs a week, and preferably one egg a day. Betty needs iron, and eggs are a useful source. Having one egg a day will add about one hundred calories. Cheese should be used to the extent of at least three ounces a week, particularly if Betty does not use the advised amount of milk. The calorie value of one ounce of Cheddar-type cheese is about 100. Betty can remain slim *and* healthy if she uses all of these essential foods in advised amounts and does *not* eat candy, cake, pastry, and does *not* use soft drinks. It is a big help to Betty to understand that she will be a better and healthier mother if she eats the essential foods during adolescence. She does need sympathetic and understanding guidance.

Habits formed in childhood persist and become more fixed as we grow older. When we help children to form good food habits we are helping them to become healthier adults with reasonable habits. The best time to start preparing for old age is in childhood. Adult life would be more interesting and healthier if we became accustomed in childhood to liking a wide variety of foods and if we developed a willingness to try new foods or even familiar foods cooked and served in new ways.

There are periods in childhood when problems of food use and food habits are particularly worth watching. The second year is one such period and this has been discussed. Another time is around the age of ten or eleven. Youngsters feel that they are growing up and becoming adult. At this time we see all too frequently the giving up of foods like milk, which are thought to be childish. If we want children to grow normally and to become healthy adults, we should be concerned about the development and preservation of good food habits as part of the general health picture.

# CHAPTER 12

# We Don't Need to Be Fat

So much has been written and said about overweight in the last few years that there may be not much left to say. On the other hand, there is still a terrific amount of confusion and misunderstanding. What follows is an attempt to set down what is known in as simple a manner as possible.

First of all, what is meant by overweight? How is overweight determined? Various tables of weight and height in respect to age are available. Older tables and some modern ones are averages for groups of people. If many people in the group are fat, the average for the group will be greater than if the majority of the group were thin. The expression, "normal weight," is used to designate these average weights. People have been considered to be overweight if their weight exceeds the normal weight plus ten per cent. To put the thing simply: suppose you are a man aged forty and your height is 5 feet 8 inches. If you look up the height-weight table which has been in use for the past forty years you will find that the "normal" weight for men of that height and age is given as 158 pounds. If you increase that by ten per cent, you get 174 pounds. If your actual weight is 180 pounds, then you are "overweight."

There are several catches in this way of deciding if people are overweight. If you look at the old, commonly used table (it will likely be labeled as coming from the Life Extension Institute and will be based on height and weight figures published in a report in 1912), you will find that "normal weights" of men and women are shown as increasing with age. To use one example, the weights of men 5 feet 8 inches are shown as increasing from 148 pounds at age twenty to 163 pounds at age fifty-five. That is what actually happens with most men but it is not what *should* happen. Not only is there no real biologic reason for increase in weight with age, but such an increase is undesirable. It happens in most people because they keep on eating as much food when they become older and less active as they did when they were young and active. It is now recognized that weight should not increase as we grow older and that we would be better if the increase did not take place.

Another difficulty in using a height-weight table is that the frame of some people is heavier than the frame of other people. Some people are stocky in build and will be heavier than slim persons of the same height. This is no proof that the stocky people are overweight. In one respect it might be better not to mention this because some people who are truly overweight claim that they are stocky in build and use that as an alibi. However, differences in body build do cause differences in weight and such differences need to be taken into account in deciding if a person is overweight.

A new type of height-weight table has come into use in recent years. It was published by the Metropolitan Life Insurance Company in 1942. Copies of the complete table are available from a number of sources. A simplified form of the table is used here. The table was prepared by considering heights and weights of people who were showing extended life expectancy. No increase in weight is regarded as desirable after twenty-five or thirty years of age. Instead of one single figure of weight for a particular height, ranges of weight for three different types of build are given (small frame, medium frame, large frame). This sounds complicated and it is complicated, unfortunately. How do you know whether to say you are small or large frame? To get away from this complication, the following simplified table is given:

DESIRABLE WEIGHTS FOR HEIGHT
*(Based on Metropolitan Life Insurance Company Statistical Bulletin No. 23, published 1942)*

| Height in Inches with shoes on | Weight in Pounds | |
| --- | --- | --- |
| | Men | Women |
| 5 feet | 112 to 138 | 104 to 128 |
| 5 feet, 2 inches | 117 to 143 | 109 to 133 |
| 5 feet, 4 inches | 121 to 149 | 115 to 141 |
| 5 feet, 6 inches | 128 to 156 | 121 to 149 |
| 5 feet, 8 inches | 135 to 165 | 128 to 156 |
| 5 feet, 10 inches | 142 to 174 | 135 to 165 |
| 6 feet | 150 to 184 | 142 to 174 |

These are wide ranges in weights. If your weight is in the lower half of the range given for your height, you may be fairly sure that your weight is desirable. If your weight is near the top of the range, you may be somewhat heavy. If your weight is above the top by more than ten pounds you are overweight.

There is another catch in deciding about overweight which does not apply to many adults. Physical training, as undergone by athletes, increases the size and weight of the muscles. Physically trained people are likely to be above desirable weight for height but not because they are fat. We are not concerned about this kind of overweight.

The kind of overweight we are concerned about is that which is brought about by an increased storage of fat in the body. This fatness is the common, garden variety of overweight. A considerable amount of fat accumulates beneath the skin. This can be evident if a fold of skin is pinched between the thumb and fingers, particularly if the fold is on the back of the upper arm, or on one side of the back midway between the shoulders and hips, or on the abdomen. There are instruments available to measure the thickness of skin folds and thus estimate the amount of fat which is in storage.

A simple, useful method is available to let you decide whether you are fat or not. Just take off your clothes and look at yourself in a mirror. After that you can decide about reading the rest of this chapter.

Why all the concern these days about overweight and fatness? There are a variety of reasons. The most important has to do with health. The records of insurance companies show that fat people are likely to die at an earlier age than slim people. Naturally, insurance companies prefer to have policyholders live as long as possible, and they don't like to sell insurance to people who are likely to die too soon. Ask any insurance company and you will be told that overweight, fat people are poor risks. Fat people may be refused an insurance policy; at least they will have difficulty in getting life insurance. Insurance companies are concerned about this because their records show that fatness is a predisposing factor leading to the development of several degenerative diseases: diabetes, gall-bladder disease, heart disease. It is in the interest of everyone to stay slim.

You are all familiar with statements about the effects of overweight on the heart in causing it to do more work. Marked overweight causes difficulties in other ways. It makes walking difficult, and fat people give up walking to just sit and store more fat. The problem of moving weight about is especially bad in people with arthritis or joint disease.

Modern taste is for slim people, and the appearance of fat people is distasteful to most of us. In one respect this is due to the example set by the modern leaders of thought and culture, the movie and television stars. Whatever the reason, anyone who now cares about appearance does not want to be fat. Women's magazines publish various special diets and the main appeal for their use is appearance. Pictures are shown of the heroine who weighed 190 pounds and was socially an outcast. By the use of the new, fabulous, banana-skin diet she got her weight down to 138 pounds, became attractive, snared a man, and is now happily married. By the time she is married for twenty years her weight will be back up unless she understands that the important reason for being slim is not appearance but health.

People put on weight, unless they are athletes in training, because they are storing fat and, to some extent, water. Fat is stored because there is more food available in the body than is needed for current expenditures of energy. Carbohydrate in excess of that needed for current energy production is converted into fat and stored as such. The body has very limited capacity for storing carbohydrate. We are not likely to have a reserve of carbohydrate greater than would meet energy needs for eighteen to twenty hours. If carbohydrate is available in greater amount, it will be stored as fat. Excess protein can be converted into fat and stored like the fat produced from carbohydrate. Excess fat in the body, coming as fat from food, will, of course, be stored as fat. The fat which accumulates in the body of a person who is becoming overweight and developing fatness does not arrive in the body by some strange miracle. It appears because there is a surplus of food, more than is needed for energy requirements. We need to realize these facts.

Of course, many fat people refuse to believe the facts. Let's consider some of the explanations which are given:

1. *"It's not what I eat—it's my glands."* The thyroid gland controls the rate of the utilization of food to furnish body heat. This portion of energy production is called basal metabolism, a term familiar to almost everyone these days and frequently considered the culprit in the production of fatness. It is true that people with an overactive thyroid have an increased rate of food utilization. It is also true that people with an underactive thyroid have a decreased rate of food utilization. Do fat people have underactive thyroids? A few do, and many do not. There are as many thin persons with underactive thyroids as there are fat people. Groups of fat and thin people have been studied in a number of clinics. In

every case, the underactive thyroids have not been found to be the general rule for fat people. A few glandular diseases do lead to overweight, but these diseases are rare.

2. *"My digestion is more efficient—I absorb more of the food I eat."* Like the gland story, this has been repeatedly investigated and the results are clear. The digestion of food in fat people is *not* more efficient than digestion in thin people. That notion is false and proved so by a mass of evidence.

3. *"Fatness runs in my family and hence I can't help it."* In some strains of rats and mice, fatness has been found to be an inherited characteristic. There is no evidence that fatness is inherited in humans. Genetic studies of fat and of thin people have shown that fatness and thinness are not inherited.

Both fatness and thinness seem to run in families but the explanation is not heredity. Children acquire eating habits from parents. If the parents are heavy eaters and are accustomed to eat until they are distended, children tend to become heavy eaters—and heavy people. There is a moral in this, if you think about it.

4. *"There is something different about the way I use foods."* This idea is often stated by a woman who says she doesn't eat any more, or even as much, as her husband and look how thin he is. If this explanation were valid it would mean that the production of energy from food constituents is super-efficient in stout people and this super-efficiency makes possible the surplus which is stored as fat. It would mean that, in comparison, the production of energy from food constituents in thin people is inefficient and wasteful so that no surplus is pos-

sible. This is a plausible story but scientific evidence does not support it. Every attempt to find a difference in the efficiency of energy production between fat and thin people has failed to provide any evidence to support this contention.

We might as well face the facts. There is only one explanation for the surplus of fat—that is, only one explanation for which there is definite, sure proof. The explanation is so simple that it is dismissed as rubbish by many stout people. The explanation: Surplus food is available to be stored as fat because the energy value of the food intake is greater than the energy expenditure. If you don't wish to accept that explanation, you can reconcile yourself to continued fatness. Unless we realize the cause we cannot appreciate the remedy or the method of prevention.

People store fat and become overweight because they eat more than they need.

Why do people eat more than needed? A variety of explanations have been offered and the main ones should be considered. The body has a mechanism which controls hunger. This mechanism was described in Chapter 1. When the amount of sugar in the blood drops to a low level, a portion of the central nervous system, close to the brain, is activated and sends a message to the stomach. Waves of contractions in the walls of the stomach give the sensation of hunger and we are prompted to eat. After the blood sugar has been increased by the absorption of sugar from eaten food, hunger ceases and we feel satisfied. In many people this mechanism operates so nicely that food intake just about equals needs. Why doesn't it operate to keep stout people from eating more than they need? It is known that an injury to the hunger-control portion of the central nervous system upsets the control and causes the eating of more food than is needed. This has been demonstrated in experimental animals but in very few humans. Another possibility is that some people use sugar very quickly and, in them, blood sugar decreases more quickly than in other people. It is guessed that stout people are fast users of sugar. The scientific studies which have been made do not support this guess.

A very likely explanation is habit. People can and do become accustomed to eating until they feel distended. After this habit is established, such people do not feel satisfied unless they have taken in enough food to make them feel distended. To them, such a feeling is a real comfort and they expect to feel like that after meals. Not only this situation, but the reverse of it, can be seen frequently. Many people have become accustomed to not feeling distended and full. When this custom is established it is just about as difficult to break as the fullness one. It is very difficult for many thin people to eat a heavy meal because they are uncomfortable if they feel full. Both attitudes toward food can develop in childhood and persist for many years. This development gives the impression that heredity is to blame, when actually attitudes toward the size of meals are acquired from parents.

We have all heard it said that stout people enjoy food. The impression is given that it is impossible to be a connoisseur of food without eating a lot. This is not true. Food can be enjoyed and savored without gluttony. If we have the habit of eating lightly, we can still enjoy good food. The flavor of a good wine can be relished by sipping a small glass—it is not necessary to drink a gallon. The pleasure of smoking a good cigar is not increased by smoking five cigars in rapid succession. Half a pound of tender, nicely cooked steak is just as appealing as two pounds.

The hunger mechanism is frequently overruled not only by personal habits but also very frequently by hospitality and social custom. Current ideas of hospitality are to put the best foot forward in serving food. Social eating is nearly as much of a menace as social drinking. But social eating doesn't get much attention. People full of alcohol can cause accidents on the way home. People full of rich cake, pastry, whipped cream, and whatnot frequently have indigestion but this doesn't damage cars or injure other people. The trouble is, of course, that social custom dictates that the host and hostess must appear to be very generous. The hostess must give the impression that she either is or has a good cook. At afternoon bridge parties women eat food when they are not hungry, food which they don't need. In the evening we have to eat large quantities of food or an unwillingness to stuff ourselves is regarded as rudeness to the hostess. We shouldn't feel it is necessary to either serve or eat 300 calories of rich cake, topped with whipped cream. It amuses me to look through women's magazines. On page 39 there will be an article on a fabulous new diet to bring about rapid weight loss. On page 65 there will be a recipe with colored illustrations of a luscious dessert, the frequent eating of which will make necessary the fabulous reducing diet. In this day and age it should not be necessary for tables to groan. It likewise should not be necessary for the partakers of hospitality to groan.

Let's go back to the question of why people overeat. Popular interest in mental health has been markedly intensified in recent years. Even some of our best movie stars find it necessary to have staff psychiatrists. The trend is to supply psychologic explanations for about everything. As a matter of course, there are now psychologic explanations for fatness. One explanation is that people gorge themselves with food to counteract a frustration. If you have been disappointed in love, or if you have not received the expected promotion, you will overeat to forget the disappointment. If your mother frustrated you by stopping you from throwing a hammer through windows, that is an alleged explanation of overeating. The frustration explanation may be valid in some cases; frustrated people do turn to alcohol as a compensation, and they might secure happiness from food. My main objection to explaining overeating on a psychologic basis is that it provides a crutch on which people can lean instead of standing firmly on their own feet. If you want to call me old-fashioned and out-of-date, go ahead.

There is a general impression that fat people are happy, contented folks and that slim people are disagreeable and unhappy. Shakespeare's Julius Caesar said: "Let me have men about me that are fat; sleek-headed men and such as sleep of night." Fat men may be happy; fat women, these days, are likely to be unhappy because of their appearance. They may have tried several reducing diets for a few days each without any visible effect. Happiness and fatness are not always found in the same person.

Let's return to the question frequently expressed by

stout persons: "I eat the same amount of food as my husband (or my wife) and look how thin he (or she) is. How do you explain that?" There are several possible explanations:

1. Is the food intake really the same, or do you just think so? All too frequently, people say that they hardly eat anything. You know the common expression: "I eat like a bird." Birds generally eat a great deal of food, perhaps more in proportion to body weight than do humans; birds are very active creatures. Fat people choose the wrong animal for the comparison. Stout people are frequently fooled about the amount of food or they try to fool others. A woman who is a good cook and fond of food may eat in the kitchen far more than she realizes. The woman who sits at a bridge table and eats a lot of candy may be fooling herself. The person who is overweight and who "eats practically nothing," will lose weight in a hospital if the food intake is really restricted.

2. However, the food intakes of the two people may have the same calorie value and body weights may be different. People deposit fat and increase in weight when the calorie intake is greater than the energy expenditure. It is readily possible to have quite different outputs of energy. One person may be energetic and active; the other may be less active. Many slim people are restless and may expend more energy than even they realize. Placid, quiet people may be quite inactive in comparison. The amount of work and the amount of exercise may be markedly different. We still come back to the one proved cause of either overweight or underweight: the balance between energy intake and energy output.

There is another point about energy output which

needs careful consideration. Energy output decreases as we grow older—our food intake should be scaled down, too. In addition, the energy expenditures of people in general have decreased in the last fifty years. At the beginning of this century a man classified as a machinist was likely to do a considerable amount of heavy, manual work. Today an operator of an automatic lathe is classified as a machinist; the amount of physical work is very different. Fifty years ago walking to work was an ordinary affair. Now, people won't walk to the corner drugstore. Some years ago, no one was alarmed about children walking two miles to school. Now they can't walk six blocks. Even the physical work on a farm has been greatly reduced. The labor of housework has been very much lessened. Men can no longer push a lawn mower; the mower must be power-operated. We can no longer carry golf clubs; we must have carts. Of course, the ultimate aim of every respectable golfer is to be moved from shot to shot in a small car. There are two comments worth making about the decrease in energy expenditure: Our food intake has not been adjusted. The average intake of calories per person per day has remained fairly constant, at least in the United States and in Canada, during the last thirty years, and possibly as far back as 1900. The second comment is the prevalence of deaths from heart disease has increased and, worse still, has spread into younger age groups. The increase has been blamed, without sound evidence, on the intake of fat. There is much better evidence relating the prevalence of heart disease to lack of exercise. Motor cars may be killing us both directly and indirectly.

Let us suppose that you feel that you are definitely overweight and are concerned about it. What should you do? The safe thing is to have a medical examination to find out whether you are actually overweight and, if so, whether you should set about losing weight and how rapidly. Attempting to lose weight quickly can be a real stress and should not be undertaken without the approval of your physician. Only he can decide whether you should attempt rapid weight reduction or whether you should go at it slowly.

If you are a housewife it is probable that your present calorie intake is somewhere between 2,000 and 2,400 a day. If you are a sedentary man your intake is likely to be 2,200-2,800 calories a day. In either case, if you are advised to lose weight rapidly, your calorie intake should be reduced to 800 a day. Slow weight reduction with less strain, less discomfort and less visible results will follow the use of an intake of 1200-1500 calories a day.

### An 800-Calorie Supply of Food

| | |
|---|---|
| 3 cups of skim milk | 260 calories |
| 1 medium orange | 70 " |
| 1 serving cabbage (raw or cooked) | 40 " |
| 1 serving cooked carrots | 44 " |
| 1 serving oatmeal porridge | 148 " |
| 1 slice enriched bread | 64 " |
| 1 serving lean meat | 197 " |
| Total | 823 calories |

This selection of foods supplies 59 grams of protein and adequate amounts of all vitamins and other nutrients needed by adults.

Possible menus for meals are:
*Breakfast:* orange, oatmeal, 1 cup milk.
*Lunch:* cabbage salad, 1 slice bread, 1 cup milk.
*Dinner:* lean beef, carrots, 1 cup milk.

Fruit, such as a peach, a small apple, or a small bunch of grapes can be added for dessert without a serious increase in calories. Clear coffee or clear tea (no cream, no sugar, but a little of the day's allotment of skim milk) can be used at any meal without an increase in calories. Several alternative foods can be used without increasing calories and without reducing nutritive value. In place of the orange there could be used one-half of a medium grapefruit, or four ounces of either orange juice or grapefruit juice or eight ounces of tomato juice. Wheat-flake porridge or one-half shredded-wheat biscuit can be used in place of oatmeal. Lettuce and tomato salad can be used in place of cabbage salad. Broccoli, cauliflower, snap beans, could be used in place of carrots. Because this 800-calorie diet is adequate with respect to all nutrients, no vitamin preparation is necessary. Dinner can be made more satisfying by adding a bit of sweetness. A small serving of sherbet (one-half a customary serving) will add sweetness at the cost of about 50 calories. Better do without this if you can.

### A 1200-Calorie Supply of Food

| | | |
|---|---:|---|
| 1 medium orange | 70 | calories |
| 1 serving oatmeal porridge | 148 | " |
| 3 slices enriched bread | 192 | " |
| 3 pats butter | 150 | " |
| 1 serving lean meat | 197 | " |
| 2 servings vegetables | | |
| (cabbage, carrots, cauliflower | 80 | " |
| 3 cups skim milk | 260 | " |
| 1 egg | 77 | " |
| Total | 1,174 | calories |

This selection of foods could be used in these meals:

*Breakfast:* orange, oatmeal, milk, 1 slice toast with butter.

*Lunch:* vegetable salad, 1 slice bread with butter, 1 egg, milk.

*Dinner:* meat, 1 vegetable, 1 slice bread with butter, milk.

Alternate foods can be used to give variety. The following alternates can be used interchangeably without appreciably altering either the calorie yield or the general nutritive value:

*Fruit:* 1 medium orange, or ½ grapefruit, or 4 ounces orange or grapefruit juice, or 4 ounces vitamin-enriched apple juice, or 8 ounces tomato juice.

*Vegetables:* cabbage, cauliflower, broccoli, snap beans, Brussels sprouts, chard, kale, turnip greens.

*Porridge:* oatmeal, wheat flakes, half a shredded-wheat biscuit

*Meat:* lean beef, lamb, lean veal, chicken, turkey, fish.

Some of the most popular foods should not be used by people who are trying to lose weight. These foods are cake, sweet cookies, pie, pastry, candy, most kinds of soft drinks, beer, and alcoholic beverages in general. All visible fat should be trimmed from meat. Skim milk should be used in place of whole milk. Butter and margarine should be restricted as much as possible.

The one real essential for weight reduction is will-power, backbone, or whatever you want to call a combination of a strong desire to lose weight, a determination to accomplish the weight reduction, and perseverance. Weight will not be lost by keeping food intake low for one day. The diet must be adhered to all day, every day, for some time. You cannot lose weight by eating no breakfast, a light lunch, and a very heavy dinner. You will not lose weight even if you stick to the diet at home and then have 800 calories at bridge in the afternoon or at a party in the evening. There is only one way to lose weight. Don't kid yourself that it can be done by lying on a vibrator couch or by sitting in a vibrator chair. Don't be a sucker for the latest fad diet or the latest reducing food.

Various drugs or preparations are sold with claims regarding appetite control. There are several drugs which will lessen hunger. They should not be used without the approval of a doctor. There are preparations which are said to lessen hunger. One type consists of squares of candy (perhaps with added vitamins). These are taken before meals. The sugar in the candy raises the blood sugar and lessens hunger. These special preparations are expensive and are no more useful than equal weights of hard candy. Why pay fancy prices for candy under another name? Do you remember P. T. Barnum? A very effective and reasonably cheap hunger-killer is a cigaret. A smoke just before a meal can lessen hunger as effectively as several expensive drugs.

Because many people know that the thyroid gland controls the rate of food utilization, and because thyroid preparations can be used to increase the rate, the doctor will be urged to prescribe thyroid tablets. For most older people a large dose of thyroid is not safe. If thyroid tablets are prescribed in a safe amount and are so taken, the rate of food utilization will be increased for a while. The person's own thyroid gland is putting out thyroid hormone but the added amount as a drug depresses the gland and less hormone is put out. The total amount (hormone from patient's gland plus that added as a drug) decreases and so does the rate of food utilization. The dose of thyroid tablets can be increased with presently the same sequence of events. There is an upper safe limit to the dose of thyroid tablets. Prescription of thyroid tablets may be a *temporary* help for a short time at the start of weight reduction but no more than that.

There is no short cut or easy method to weight reduction. The only sure way is to reduce the intake of calories. What about increasing calorie expenditure by exercise? The energy expenditure in ordinary types of exercise is much less than is commonly thought. A walk of two miles at an ordinary pace is a long walk for us moderns. Such a walk expends the energy supplied by two slices of bread and butter; some people would find it easier not to eat the bread. Outdoor exercise tends to increase hunger and that can lead to departing from the reducing diet. This is not an argument against exercise; most of us would do better to have exercise, suitable for our age, every day. But don't let's fool ourselves that we can lose a lot of weight by exercise.

After we have followed an 800-calorie diet for a few weeks we will realize that prevention is much better than treatment. People who are slim should eat to stay slim. It is useful to start the prevention of fatness in childhood and certainly in adolescence.

Fatness is the most prevalent nutrition problem in the United States and in Canada. Fatness is a health problem. Fat people don't look nice. Fatness can be prevented by eating sensibly—see Chapter 11 for the kind of meals to eat to stay slim.

# CHAPTER | 13

## *As We Grow Older*

An old truism, often repeated, is that the main needs of older people are less work, more warmth, and less food. It may seem strange but these three needs can be tied together and the use of food is a common factor.

If we calculate energy production per pound of body weight so that the amount of energy production can be compared from one person to another and even compared for children and adults, we find that energy production per pound of weight is greatest at the end of the first year of life. From then on there is a continuous slow decrease. Energy production at age seventy is less than at sixty and that, in turn, is less than at fifty. The changes can be expressed clearly in calories.

*Average Daily Calorie Expenditures*
*for Adults of Average Weight*

| Age | Man 150 lbs. | Woman 125 lbs. |
|---|---|---|
| 25 | 3200 | 2200 |
| 45 | 3000 | 2050 |
| 65 | 2550 | 1750 |

In addition to the gradual decrease in energy production for the maintenance of the body, most people become less active as they grow older and consequently expend less energy for work and exercise. Total energy needs (as shown above) decrease with age and hence the need for food (as expressed in calories) is lessened. Less work and less food tie together.

The need for more warmth may be tied to food in two ways. As we grow older the body burns less food to produce heat. We need to live in a warmer environment. This may mean keeping the house warmer and wearing heavier clothing. As a general rule there is a feeling of warmth after eating owing to an increase in energy production. The increase is temporary and is produced particularly by the eating of protein. This feeling of warmth, even though it is temporary, gives comfort to older people. It can be brought about by eating meals which contain a fair amount of protein.

As has been pointed out, the need for calories decreases with age. The needs for protein, iron, calcium and various vitamins do *not* lessen. Special attention should be given to protein. There is a continuous loss of protein from body tissues throughout life and the loss must be made good to prevent wastage. High-quality protein is obtained from meat, milk, eggs, fish, poultry, cheese. Older people may not be able to chew meat. They may not be able to afford some or all of these protein-rich foods. Of these foods, milk and cheese are the most economical sources of protein. If older people are living alone, they may be unable to cook or they may not bother to cook. All of these circumstances may reduce the intake of protein—such a reduction is undesirable from the viewpoint of both health and comfort. As we grow older we should give particular attention to the use of these foods:

*Milk:* We should have at least ½ pint and preferably 1 pint a day. This will help our intakes of protein, calcium and riboflavin. Money can be saved by using skim milk made by adding the right amount of skim-milk powder to the proper amount of water. If we don't want to drink milk (which is a pity), it can be used in making soup, or porridge, and in custard desserts. If little milk is used cheese should be eaten, at least 1 ounce a day. Cheese is a cheap source of protein and calcium.

*Fruit:* We should have 1 medium orange, or ½ grapefruit, or 4 ounces of orange or grapefruit juice, or 8 ounces of tomato juice every day to supply ascorbic acid. In addition one other fruit should be used daily.

*Vegetables:* We should have a small serving of potatoes and we should have two other vegetables every day. These vegetables should be cooked until they are just tender enough to eat but not overcooked.

*Meat, Fish, Fowl:* One serving of one of these foods should be eaten every day.

*Bread and Cereal:* Three to four slices of bread a day will be sufficient. A serving of breakfast cereal with the nutritive value of whole grain should be used.

This list of foods, in the quantities described, will supply about 1,700 calories, a suitable amount for older people. It should be noted that the daily use of these foods in the right amounts will ensure adequate amounts of protein and of all essential nutrients, *including vitamins*. If we use these foods as described, no vitamin preparation will be necessary, or advisable.

As we grow older, our digestive apparatus becomes less active. It may not be possible to eat certain foods which can be eaten by younger people without difficulty. Some people have digestive difficulty with corn and it can be omitted. Pickles, spices, and high-seasoned foods are undesirable for older persons. Foods fried in fat often cause indigestion and should be on the banned list. Constipation often becomes a problem and can develop into an obsession. It is very wise to consult a doctor about constipation and not to attempt treatment without medical advice. The cause may be quite different from what you think. Bran is a popular laxative. Unfortunately, it can cause irritation in some persons, at least. There are two measures which are generally safe to help prevent constipation. One is a generous intake of water. The other is a generous intake of foods providing bulk in a softened, non-irritating form. A number of cooked vegetables and fruits will do this.

The slowing-down of digestive arrangements makes a change in meal size advisable. It is better for older people to spread food more evenly through the day and avoid a big, hearty meal. It is a good idea to reduce the load on the digestive tract. A more substantial breakfast, a bigger lunch or supper, and a smaller dinner help to give freedom from indigestion and hence is more comfortable.

Many people sleep better if they feel comfortable when they go to bed and do not feel hungry. A large proportion of older people feel better if they have a bedtime snack. This may include a glass of milk or a cup of cocoa with a cookie. Sometimes fruit can be used.

Food habits and food notions can be decidedly rigid and they can keep older people from eating foods needed for health. Frequently oranges and grapefruit will be refused because of the notion that the acid in these fruits causes rheumatism. We can try to explain that the fruit acid is turned into a base in the body and this base neutralizes acid from other sources but, very often, the explanation comes up against a stone wall of fixed notions. Some older people are sure that they should not eat meat because it is harmful to elderly people. If people have been unaccustomed to drinking milk, they are not likely to start a new habit. Arguing about these matters or even trying to provide a reasonable explanation can be a waste of time. If you are concerned with the care of an older person, it is better to try subterfuges. Citrus fruit or citrus juice may be refused at breakfast; citrus fruit can be used for dessert and accepted, especially if the acid flavor is masked with a bit of sugar. Milk can be used on porridge and considerable quantities of milk can be used in cooking, as can cheese.

In recent years the proportion of older people in the population of the United States and Canada has increased. The main reason has been the lengthening of the life span and the control of some infectious diseases which formerly caused the death of children. Compulsory retirement plans are now nearly universal and there has developed considerable concern about the welfare of older people. Nutrition is not only one of the factors which control health; it has, also, real influence on comfort and contentment.

In any large community there are likely to be a considerable number of older people living alone, often in single rooms. Facilities for cooking are meager and there is little incentive for cooking. There isn't much pleasure in eating alone. Financial problems frequently exist. Pensions may be small. Buying food for one person is not as economical as buying for a family. Storage arrangements may be poor and food wastage may add to the expense of eating.

At least two types of service are developing in communities to help older people to have better meals. One arrangement is to distribute meals prepared in a central kitchen. Distribution is made by truck. This procedure counteracts the problems of purchasing for one person and of cooking for one person. The procedure does not deal with the unpleasantness of eating alone. Another obvious aspect is that food prepared in a central kitchen and kept warm for some time may not taste as good as food prepared just before eating. It is difficult to keep such food from having an "institutional" flavor and appearance.

A second procedure is to have community eating. This may or may not give more appealing meals; it can give sociability and company. Moreover, the meal service can be combined with light work activities which keep life from becoming monotonous and which make older people feel that they are still useful. In one such arrangement, older people come to a central house in the morning, carry on light activities, have a good noon meal, designed to ensure that they will have at least one substantial meal in the day, and continue with some activity in the afternoon. In addition to obtaining a good meal, the older people can get out of their rooms, meet others, and chat.

Many of the eating problems of older people could have been prevented by the formation of good habits in childhood. When parents encourage children to use food healthfully, they are doing far more than seeing that children get food needed for growth. Attitudes toward food tend to persist through life and to become more and more rigid. Preparation for old age should start in childhood.

# CHAPTER 14

# *Food Nonsense Is a Nuisance*

Everyone would agree that the sum of two plus two is four. This is a nice, simple, and definite statement with which there will not be any disagreement. In no community will we find a notion, passed on from one generation to the next, that two plus two equals five. It is not possible to buy a book written by an alleged expert who has not studied arithmetic which sets out to prove to the reader that two plus two equals three. Manufacturers of building blocks do not claim in advertising that their blocks can be used to prove that two plus two equals either three or five. Moreover, no government regulation will be necessary to stop such advertising.

A tremendous difference exists between arithmetic and nutrition. With regard to foods and their use there is a vast amount of confusion. Conflicting statements are common. Notions, approaching folklore in nature, are passed around about commonly used foods. These notions are believed by many people, and foods good to eat and good for health are not eaten. Fad diets claimed to cause people to lose weight or to prevent certain diseases are published in newspapers or in magazines. Because they appear in print they are accepted as valuable, particularly by those who have graduated from colleges or universities. Instead of getting suitable medical care, people take up fads, either for a diet or for special foods. A number of books, written by self-described experts, are available to provide misinformation. Some of these "experts" give lectures, particularly to women's clubs; no one seems to worry whether the "experts" know anything about the subject. All sorts of misleading statements are attempted in advertising foods and drugs, and government officials in food and drug laboratories must be continuously on the alert to keep the public protected.

In this chapter an attempt will be made to discuss fallacious notions and fads. It will not be possible to do this completely. Notions vary from one community to another and the writer does not claim to know all of the various notions. Some of the more frequently encountered fads will be considered. In addition, there will be given some simple criteria which can be used to tell whether an "expert" knows anything about the subject of nutrition.

### Notions

Some of the erroneous notions about food are found only in certain communities; in other cases the notions are widespread. Some of them have been in existence for several generations, at least, while others are fairly modern.

Several notions about milk are encountered frequently. A common one is that milk is all right for babies and young children but should not be used by adults. At any age, milk is an economical source of high-quality protein, of calcium, and of the vitamin riboflavin. All of these nutrients are needed *throughout* life. Moreover, milk is easily digested. Doctors use milk as the main food in a number of special diets because it is easily digested and well tolerated. Milk is claimed to cause phlegm in the throat; there is no sound reason for this notion. One of the worst notions about milk is that it causes cancer. Neither milk nor any other food will cause cancer. This absurd story about milk is spread by people with evangelistic fervor. It has been claimed that the pasteurization of milk seriously lessens its nutritive value. There is clear proof that pasteurized milk will give the same rate of growth in children as will raw milk. The pasteurization of milk is a valuable method to prevent the spread of several infectious diseases and pasteurization of milk should be compulsory.

Almost everyone has heard it said that cheese is difficult to digest and that it causes constipation. Careful tests of the digestibility of most common foods have been made and it has been shown that cheese is digested easily—even by children of three or four years. There is no truth in the notion that cheese causes constipation. That notion is a ridiculous libel on a very palatable, healthful, and economical food. The bad feature of this notion is that it keeps gullible people from eating cheese.

Some people refuse to eat oranges because they think that the fruit acid is bad for rheumatism. It is hard to convince these people that the fruit acid is converted to a base (the opposite of an acid) in the body and that the base neutralizes acids from other sources. The amusing aspect of it is that some of them will eat oranges with added sugar because they can't taste the acid—it's still there but masked by the sugar.

Another notion which is held by some older people these days is that meat is harmful because a liberal eating of meat is said to damage the liver and kidneys. About fifty years ago a scientist in the United States, Russell Chittenden, believed that a large intake of protein would be harmful for the same reason. It has been shown that people can adapt themselves and maintain health on protein intakes varying between thirty and three hundred grams a day. Observations of Eskimos have established that people can adapt themselves to very large intakes of meat without any harmful effects. Adherence to this notion by older people is unfortunate because refusal to eat meat deprives them of a source of needed protein and of essential vitamins and iron.

The evangelistic fervor with which a number of people urge that everyone eat whole wheat bread has subsided considerably. It is true that whole wheat bread has a better nutritive value than white bread, even when the white bread is made with "enriched" flour. If people use proper amounts of milk, eggs, meat, the nutritive value of the bread is not important because the nutrients contained in whole wheat bread will be supplied by other foods. In areas in which milk, eggs, meat, are scarce and where grain foods are used in large amounts, the nutritive value of those grain products is important.

Some twenty years ago, experiments on rabbits showed that the inclusion of considerable amounts of cholesterol in the food given the rabbits caused changes in the arteries which looked like atherosclerosis in humans.

From these experiments, it was assumed that people who wished to avoid coronary heart disease should restrict the use of foods containing appreciable quantities of cholesterol. One such food is eggs and advice was provided that people should stop eating eggs. The advice should not have been given for several reasons. Rabbits are herbivorus animals, accustomed to live on green food which never contains cholesterol—rabbits are unaccustomed to food containing cholesterol and the utilization of this substance is not the same in rabbits as it is in humans. In recent years cholesterol has been portrayed as a villain—we have been told that a high content of cholesterol in the blood causes changes in the arteries which are conducive to the production of coronary heart disease. No step in this sequence of events has yet been proven. Cholesterol serves a number of very useful purposes in the body and it could properly be described as an essential substance. The body can and does make cholesterol from starch and sugar; the amount of cholesterol produced in the body increases when the intake of cholesterol in the foods is decreased. Even if it were proven that a high content of cholesterol in the blood is harmful (which is guessed at but not proven), the amount of cholesterol in the food we eat has very little effect on the amount of cholesterol in the blood because of the production of cholesterol in the body. There is no good reason for not eating eggs. There are several good reasons *for* eating eggs: they are appetizing, healthful food—good sources of protein, iron, various vitamins. The supposed reason for refusing to eat eggs has no more scientific support than many of the folklore notions.

Have you heard the notion about parsnips becoming poisonous if they are left in the ground all winter and start to sprout in the spring? This notion seems to be prevalent around the Great Lakes. Leaving parsnips in the ground during the winter is a handy method of storage. When they sprout some of the starch in them turns to sugar and the parsnips are much sweeter. On the basis of personal experience, I can assure you that sprouted parsnips are not only safe to eat—they are very tasty.

Various combinations of food are held to be harmful. For instance, the use of milk or ice cream in a meal with a lobster is thought to be dangerous. Whenever I am fortunate enough to have a lobster, I always order ice cream for dessert. Waiters in restaurants in various cities have refused to serve the ice cream. It would be interesting to know how this notion got started. Perhaps the original observation came as a consequence of eating either a bad lobster or infected ice cream; either one, by itself, could have caused illness. Sanitation and methods of storing and shipping foods have improved in recent years so that both lobsters and ice cream are safer than they were fifty years ago.

There is a widespread notion, deliberately fostered in some books and publications, that fruits and vegetables grown with the aid of "natural" fertilizers (like manure) are more healthful than if a chemical fertilizer is used. This seems to be part of a cult about "natural" foods. Dr. Maynard, of Cornell University, was asked by the American Medical Association to review all of the evidence regarding the differences resulting from the use of natural fertilizers as against chemical fertilizers. Dr. Maynard reported that there was no good evidence that natural fertilizers produced more healthful foods than did chemical fertilizers. The whole cult of "natural" foods is a curious one. It is hard to get a precise explanation of what is meant by the term, "natural foods." Refined sugar is apparently not a natural food and hence is harmful. The notion that food processing or food preservation is harmful is prevalent, often without sound reason. Canned vegetables can, and frequently do, have better nutritive value than the so-called fresh vegetables sold in stores. Vegetables can lose appreciable nutritive value during shipping and storage. In order to have good appearance and good flavor in products, commercial canners make great efforts to can vegetables in as fresh a condition as possible, before the vegetables have lost flavor, appearance, and nutritive value. Hence the value of canned vegetables may be better than that of a vegetable bought some days after harvesting. If we followed the natural food cult we would eat wheat as is and refrain from eating bread. Bread is a wholesome and economical food. It would be silly to eat wheat and refuse bread.

### Fad Diets

A fad diet is a set of menus advocated generally by people who have little or no knowledge of nutrition, but sometimes recommended on the basis of inadequate evidence by nutritionists. Fad diets may stress either the absence or the presence of particular foods or combinations of foods. Fad diets are recommended most often to accomplish weight reduction. Fad diets have short lives and persons who are addicted to dietary fads shift from one to another with considerable rapidity. Very often fad diets are advised for the prevention or alleviation of a disease. They exist because of a combination of ignorance and gullibility. People will clutch at almost any straw to regain health. For many generations there have been passing waves of enthusiasm for the teachings of those who have advised special diets to cure diseases.

A very celebrated diet for loss of weight was recommended almost one hundred years ago. In 1863 William Banting, in England, published "A Letter on Corpulence Addressed to the Public." Banting had been greatly overweight and, after numerous attempts to lose weight, he finally adopted a special diet which did cause him to lose considerable weight. He was so pleased with the result that he published the details of the diet and strongly recommended its use. The Banting diet contained meat, fish and fruit. For breakfast he ate about four ounces of meat or fish and not more than one ounce of toast. Dinner at noon consisted of a more liberal serving of meat, fruit, vegetables other than potatoes and an ounce of toast. For afternoon tea Banting had a rusk and a small amount of fruit. Supper in the evening consisted only of four ounces of meat or fish. Tea without milk or sugar was used and each day Banting had several glasses of either sherry or claret. It is worth noting that the Banting diet was high in protein and in this respect resembled several modern dietary fads. The main charactristic of the Banting diet was that it had a daily calorie value of about 1,400. It is likely that the meals Banting used before the diet was started supplied 2,500-3,000 calories. The marked reduction in the intake of calories, and not any virtue of a special combination of foods, was responsible for the loss of weight.

Any special diet which markedly reduces the calorie intake will cause a loss in weight. It is not wise to use a special diet which does not meet the needs for protein and all essential nutrients. Most of the reducing diets which are advocated from time to time fail to meet health specifications. There are several features about following fad diets which actually turn out to be beneficial. Many of the diets are so different from customary food intakes and are so unpleasant to follow that they are used for only short periods—generally not long enough to produce the nutrient deficiencies which would be inevitable if the diet were used for some months. People who take up fad diets skip from one to another with considerable speed and this may save them from the deficiency states. A number of the special reducing diets are recommended only for short periods; they are taken up in the hope that weight will be lost quickly and will stay lost. The major difficulty is that the diet is followed for a few weeks, some weight is lost, the person wearies of well-doing and goes right back to former habits. The weight comes back on.

Many of these fad reducing diets are just plain silly. One example is the various fruit diets. About the first of these was "the grape diet," consisting of grapes and toast. Another variation was a diet of oranges and a small amount of toast. More recently, there has been a lemon juice diet. To take the orange diet as an example of these fruit diets, a person following it will eat ten oranges a day and perhaps two slices of dry toast. The calorie value will be about twelve hundred a day. Such a calorie intake will bring about a loss in weight. The total amount of protein secured will be about one half of the minimal amount needed for the maintenance of health; obviously there will be trouble if the orange diet is continued for more than a few days.

In the past few years high-fat reducing diets have been advocated. We have been told to use cream, butter and the fat from meat liberally and promises are made that we will lose weight and feel much healthier. Other sources of advice urge that the intake of fat, particularly from animal sources, be sharply reduced to prevent coronary heart disease. It's quite a dilemma, isn't it? If we put the two types of advice together, we will eat a lot of fat, lose weight but die suddenly of coronary thrombosis. Oh well, if we smoke heavily at the same time we will develop lung cancer. Life is getting to be difficult, at least if we pay attention to various current beliefs. To go back to high-fat reducing diets. In some people such a diet has caused a loss of weight because the diet has been found sufficiently unpalatable that only a reduced portion of food has been eaten. The high content of fat has no particular virtue in regard to health.

Fad diets have been advocated for reasons other than weight reduction. There have been fads which were supposed to prevent or cure diseases or to give better health and vigor. In some cases sales of special health foods were involved. Some years ago there was a diet which depended on ignorance of the functions of the digestive system. It was advocated by a William Howard Hay and it became known as the Hay diet—but it was not intended for horses. Hay argued that the digestive tract was not able to digest carbohydrate and protein at the same time. He said that people should eat "carbohydrate meals" free of protein and "protein meals" free of carbohydrate. If Hay had been right a number of common foods should not be eaten. Bread and potatoes contain both carbohydrate and protein. Hay had other intriguing diet notions: it was wrong to drink water with meals; it paid to fast for a day or two occasionally. Of course, the basic idea that carbohydrate and protein cannot be digested and absorbed when eaten together was without any truth. Unfortunately, it was believed by a considerable number of gullible people.

Reference has been made earlier in this chapter to the notion that eggs should not be eaten because they contain cholesterol. Low-cholesterol diets became very fashionable and, in some quarters, are still thought to be useful for the prevention of heart disease.

Perhaps the worst dietary fad in recent years has been the low-fat food intake claimed to prevent coronary heart disease. This fad was launched about the time of President Eisenhower's highly publicized heart attack. It claimed that coronary heart disease was prevalent in the United States because the intake of fat was very generous. It was noted that both the prevalence of heart disease and the proportion of fat in meals was much less in Japan than in the United States. Careful consideration of the information from twelve countries convinced Dr. Hilleboe, Commissioner of Health for New York State, that the prevalence of coronary heart disease did not keep pace with fat intake in these twelve countries. Fat intake is reasonably uniform in various states in the U.S.A.; the prevalence of deaths from coronary heart disease is anything but uniform in various sections of the country. It is now apparent that a number of factors are involved in the production of coronary heart disease. Two factors have been established as being concerned in the process: obesity and lack of exercise. Men who exercise or do physical work regularly are less likely to have a coronary attack and, if they do have such an attack, it will be less severe than in men who do not exercise or do physical work. Marked fatness is a predisposing factor in the development of heart disease—and of other diseases. There is as yet no clear evidence relating the type of food intake, either in total fat or in kind of fat, to the production of coronary heart disease. In a report published in October, 1958, the U.S. Food and Nutrition Board summed up the situation with these sentences:

"The causes and course of the development of atheroma in man are still unknown.

"The question of how much and what kind of fat we should eat remains unanswered.

"Until it is clearer which fats are more desirable nutritionally and which, if any, are undesirable, major changes in American dietary habits are not to be recommended."

The moral of the craze for reducing fat intake to prevent heart disease is that jumping on a band wagon can be hazardous—it's a nasty fall off the other side.

### Stumping the "Experts"

One hundred years ago in England Banting established himself as an authority on reducing diets. There have been many similar situations since then. In the last thirty years there have been a succession of persons writing newspaper articles, magazine articles, and books about what to eat. The majority of these persons have had no training in science and, more particularly, in nutrition. In addition to income from writing, some of these people have profited from the sale of special foods or of drug preparations.

Many of you will recall the man who was especially popular about ten years ago, who had his name on several books, and who gave lectures. Hauser advocated the generous use of wheat germ, yoghurt and crude molasses. This combination was said to prevent or cure a variety of diseases and to give marvelous health. These three foods are satisfactory enough but they do not possess, either singly or in combination, the virtues which were claimed.

Following in his wake was another expert, Lelord Kordel, who also had his name on several books, who gave lectures, and was responsible for syndicated articles in newspapers. The history of this man was most interesting. Claims were made that he possessed a degree of Doctor of Science. One newspaper stated that the degree had been given by a British university. On another occasion the degree was said to have been obtained at the University of California. Actually, the man has had no significant degree of formal training in science. On a number of occasions, United States courts have condemned "health" products he has sponsored. This "expert" urged people to eat millet and sunflower seeds to obtain protein. Of course, eggs, milk, meat, cheese, fish, fowl, are much better sources of protein. However, millet and sunflower seeds were claimed to have special health merits.

An interesting example of the presentation of information is the book, *Let's Eat Right to Keep Fit,* by Adelle Davis. The title of Chapter 16 in that book is one which I quote with relish, "A Plea for Caution and Open-Mindness." This chapter is devoted to an alleged relation between B vitamins and heart disease. Over a page is occupied with a list of famous men who died of heart disease and who, it is claimed, would have lived twenty to thirty years longer if they had had an adequate intake of B vitamins. I quote from the bottom of page 125 of the book: "I recently watched another seemingly healthy man who sneered at the idea of adequate nutrition and whose requirements for the B vitamins were extremely high; some ten days after I had predicted that he could not live long, he died of heart disease."

It is true that severe deficiencies of thiamine ( a B vitamin) can bring about changes in the heart and heart failure; this condition is rarely found in the United States, in Canada, and in Great Britain. The notion that B vitamin deficiencies are common and cause heart disease is not valid. In this connection it is wise to recall a statement made by Dr. J. M. Ruffin, a distinguished American clinician: "Vitamins are not the panacea of all ills; they afford little relief in social, financial or domestic problems, long-continued treatment with expensive vitamins is a serious and unnecessary drain on the patient's pocket-book and, in the last analysis, a well-balanced diet is the best treatment in most of the cases of mild vitamin deficiencies."

However, some of you may be concerned with a practical application of the heart disease claim made by Adelle Davis. How would you know if you were deficient in B vitamins? Fortunately the necessary information is available in the book in question, but not in the same chapter. On page 113 is advice to take powdered yeast to supply B vitamins; people are advised to take small doses and gradually increase the amount. I quote from page 113: "One reason for taking yeast in small amounts at first is that, in case your digestion is faulty, yeast may blow you up like a Zeppelin. Since faulty digestion is usually the result of inadequate B vitamins, the more gas you get from yeast, the more deficient you can know that you are in B vitamins, and the more you need the yeast."

Let's combine Chapter 16 and page 113 of the Adelle Davis book in a simple manner. Take a good-sized dose of yeast. If you have a large amount of gas, you are deficient in B vitamins and are likely to die of heart disease shortly. This is so simple and practical that it is a pity that it is not supported by scientific evidence. That lack doesn't really matter, except to skeptical people. Think of the advertising possibilities—"Take Our Yeast to See If You Will Die of Heart Disease." I am surprised that there hasn't been a magazine article entitled, "Yeast, Gas, and Heart Disease."

It should be noted that indigestion can be caused by a number of factors; the relation of B vitamins to digestion is doubtful. The causes of heart disease are not known. The quotations from the book, *Let's Eat Right to Keep Fit,* are illustrative of a considerable amount of misinformation.

How can you find out whether the "experts" and the writers are authentic or phonies? There is one simple test: If claims are made that particular foods or combinations of foods are related to either the production or the prevention of cancer, arthritis, heart disease, or several other diseases, or that particular foods will give a super level of health, you can assume at once that the experts or writers are unreliable and should be received skeptically. Don't be gullible enough to believe everything that gets into print.

Sometimes very elegant names will be used for organizations which are said to support the "experts" or their statements. Reputable organizations will not lend their names or prestige for such purposes. If a book is endorsed by an officer of an organization with a resounding name, you should be skeptical. To help you in sorting out authentic from phony organizations here is a list of ones which are completely authentic and reliable and which have a genuine interest in the science of nutrition:

*In the U.S.A.* — American Medical Association
American Public Health Association
American Institute of Nutrition (there is an organization with a somewhat similar name which is not truly a scientific outfit).
American Dietetic Association
American Home Economics Association

*In Canada* — Canadian Medical Association
Canadian Public Health Association
Nutrition Society of Canada
Canadian Dietetic Association
Canadian Home Economics Association

*In Britain* — British Medical Association
The Nutrition Society

There are simple ways of getting information as to whether an "expert," or a writer, or a lecturer (on nutrition or dietetics) is authentic. Inquiries can be made to your physician, to your medical officer of health, or to a public health nurse. If they do not have the answer available immediately, they can get it. Reliable information can be obtained from government food and drug laboratories and from medical associations. The American Home Economics Association has published an excellent leaflet on food fads and nonsense.

No person who has proper scientific training can promise the super level of health, the freedom from disease, or the cures claimed by the phony experts or by some of the popular writers.

## Advertising

In several countries there are regulations regarding claims which can legally be made in advertising and in labeling. The enforcement is the responsibility of government food-and-drug officials. The regulations and the enforcing agencies merit every bit of support that we can give them. They are working to keep foods and drugs safe and to prevent fraud. It is in the interest of everyone—including manufacturers—that the work be encouraged and supported. It would be difficult to find a group more dedicated to public service or more selfless. If you suspect fraudulent claims or are uneasy about the safety of a product, it pays to get in touch with a food-and-drug official.

Despite the best efforts, the policing of advertising and of claims on labels is a difficult job. Deceptive statements and claims are attempted repeatedly. At present considerable claims are being made about the protein in breakfast cereals. In all cases of which I am aware the protein in the cereal is *not* high-quality protein. The cereal protein is markedly improved in combination with the protein of the milk usually put on the cereal. The same is true of bread-and-milk. However, the advertising for these cereals gives the impression that protein is a scarce nutrient and that many people need protein so much that they should eat the advertised cereal. In the highly developed countries excellent sources of high-quality protein are readily available. The average intake of protein per person in the United States, in Canada, and in Britain is about double actual need.

It pays to look at advertising for drugs with a critical

eye. Not all printed statements are true, just because they are in print. The advertising claims made even by the high-salaried TV personality are not necessarily reliable.

# CHAPTER 15

# *Food or Pills?*

At least six vitamins are needed by humans for normal functions in the body and hence to attain and maintain health. Chronic deficiencies of some of these cause specific diseases—diseases now seldom seen in highly developed countries. There is scientific information about minimal needs for the vitamins and, also, for other nutrients. There is a notion that, if something is good, a lot of it is much better. That notion does not hold for the vitamins or for other nutrients. If we have intakes sufficient to meet our needs, excess intakes will not give extra benefits to our health. The benefits will accrue to people who make and sell vitamin preparations but not to the consumer.

Large excesses of two of the vitamins can be harmful. These two are A and D. Babies, children, teen-agers, and expectant mothers need 400 units of vitamin D a day. Some years ago Dr. Philip Jeans, a distinguished pediatrician, reported that some babies would be harmed by intakes of 2,000 units of vitamin D a day. That statement has been amply verified by experience. Within the past few years there have been repeated occurrences of illness in babies who were getting 2,000-2,500 units of vitamin D a day. In the first few years after highly concentrated preparations of vitamin D became available, some babies were killed by administration of excessive amounts of the vitamin.

Excess quantities of vitamins and other nutrients which are soluble in water (vitamins A and D are insoluble in water) are excreted in the urine. Scurvy is caused by a prolonged lack of ascorbic acid (vitamin C). Experiments on humans have been made to find out how much ascorbic acid is needed to prevent scurvy. It has been found that ten milligrams of ascorbic acid a day will prevent scurvy and that thirty milligrams a day is sufficient for health. If a large dose of ascorbic acid is taken, the amount in excess of actual need is excreted in the urine within a few hours. To make this practical it should be noted that a medium-sized orange or half a grapefruit will supply an adult's need for ascorbic acid for a day. There is no evidence that intakes of ascorbic acid in excess of need will make people any healthier or any freer of disease.

To make matters worse, silly and unfounded claims are made about ascorbic acid. It is said to prevent the common cold, hay fever, asthma, heart disease, or at least to moderate attacks of some of these diseases. No sure method of preventing a cold has yet been devised. Ample evidence is available that large doses of any vitamin or any combination of vitamins will not prevent colds or moderate them. There is no decent evidence that ascorbic acid is useful in preventing any disease or in treating any disease except scurvy—and that effect is proved.

Are you tired? Do you want to prevent "winter ills"? Advertising claims state that taking vitamin preparations will do the trick—they won't. In recent years people in the United States, in Canada, in Britain, and elsewhere have spent millions in buying unnecessary vitamin preparations. Manufacturers of vitamin preparations and drugstores have benefited; the consumers have not benefited.

If foods are selected with sense, adequate amounts of all essential nutrients (except vitamin D) can be obtained by eating appetizing and healthful meals. Vitamin D is needed by babies, children, adolescents, and expectant mothers during the second half of pregnancy. We have no evidence that adults, other than pregnant women, need vitamin D or will benefit from a supply of this vitamin. The common notion that vitamin D will prevent colds is not true.

There are people who enjoy taking pills. For such people, vitamin pills have a mental effect. The taking of pills gives them the impression that they are looking after themselves. Of course, there are people who are chronic invalids and who seem to enjoy being sick or assuming that they are sick. There is one sound bit of advice: if you don't feel well, see your doctor. Don't try to doctor yourself because the treatment may be useless or it may be harmful. Harm can result from not having the proper treatment.

The place to buy vitamins is the food store, in foods, and not the drugstore. Unless you get enjoyment from taking pills, you should be able to enjoy good meals. If the meals include a wide variety of foods, they will be interesting and attractive, and they are likely to give you all needed nutrients, including vitamins.

A great deal is said about extra needs for various nutrients during pregnancy. Some needs are increased. In the second half of pregnancy it is advisable to increase the intake of protein, of calcium, and of iron. All three nutrients can be secured easily from foods which are readily available. A pint of milk a day, in addition to customary use, will furnish the extra protein and calcium. If it is advisable not to increase body weight, skim milk should be used. Calcium tablets are more expensive than milk as a source of calcium and the tablets, unlike milk, will not provide protein and other essential nutrients. An adequate supply of iron can be obtained from meat, eggs, and vegetables. If there is any doubt about what should be done in pregnancy, the advice of a physician should be sought *and followed.*

The notion that vitamin D or any other vitamin will prevent colds by giving a super state of resistance is part of a general belief that a lot is better than some. A deficiency—that is, an intake less than need—of any nutrient is likely to lower resistance to infection. When the deficiency is corrected, resistance to infection is brought back to the normal level. There is absolutely no evidence that resistance can be made abnormal by taking an excess of any nutrient.

Other unfounded claims have been made about various vitamins. The administration of extra thiamine (one of the B vitamins) has been said to improve the learning ability of children. A report of a test of extra thiamine on a group of children is cited as proof. There were odd features about the results of the test. The children given extra thiamine apparently showed improved learning ability in addition but not in subtraction. They also had improved vision in one eye but not in the other. If you want to believe that sort of stuff, go ahead.

In recent years there have been several extravagant claims about vitamin E. This vitamin is needed by several species of animals. Because vitamin E is necessary for normal pregnancy in rats, it was used for a while to attempt to prevent premature termination of pregnancy. The big excitement developed when it was reported that large doses would prevent heart disease. The claim petered out and was followed by stories about beneficial effects of vitamin E in diabetes and in cancer. Up to the present, there is no evidence that vitamin E is needed by humans. Moreover, we have not any evidence that vitamin E serves any useful purpose in the human body. It cannot be classed, at present, as an essential nutrient for humans.

Wheat germ oil contains a great deal of vitamin E and there is at present on the market a preparation of wheat germ oil which is claimed to do wonders. In the past few weeks I saw an advertisement for wheat germ oil in a well-known magazine. The advertisement claimed that taking wheat germ oil would produce a marvelous state of vigor. I don't believe it.

Drug preparations containing nutrients other than vitamins are available and are advertised extensively. Mention has been made of calcium tablets which are sometimes recommended for pregnant women. Preparations containing iron are advertised frequently. Adequate amounts of iron—at least sufficient for normal persons—can be secured easily from foods.

The statements made in this chapter about vitamins and other preparations may not be applicable to persons who have had severe deficiencies and who are under medical care. In such cases it may be advisable to give large doses for a few days to speed recovery. However, even cases of severe deficiencies recover remarkably well on smaller amounts supplied by foods. The notion has been encouraged by some vitamin manufacturers that very large doses are necessary for people to recover from deficient states. Actual experience has shown repeatedly that amounts supplied by good meals are generally sufficient, even with deficient patients.

Several times in this chapter the statement has been made that adequate quantities of all essential vitamins, with the exception of vitamin D, can be obtained by eating foods. To show you how this can be done, the following list gives the quantities of some foods which can be used to provide the needs of a normal man for one day:

*Vitamin A:* 2 ounces of cooked diced carrots, *or* 2 ounces of cooked spinach, *or* 3 ounces of baked winter squash, *or* 2 ounces of cooked turnip greens, *or* one-half of a small sweet potato baked, *or* 1 ounce of cooked liver.

*Thiamine:* 6 ounces baked ham, *or* 2 average pork chops, *or* a combination of 3 cups milk *plus* 4 slices enriched white bread *plus* 1 boiled potato *plus* a serving of oatmeal porridge.

*Riboflavin:* 1 pint milk *or* 2 ounces cooked liver.

*Niacin:* 2 ounces cooked liver, *or* 3 ounces roast beef *plus* 4 slices enriched white bread *plus* 1 boiled potato, *or* 1 pork chop *plus* 4 slices enriched white bread *plus* 1 serving canned peas.

*Ascorbic Acid:* 1 medium orange, *or* ½ grapefruit, *or* 4 ounces of orange juice, *or* 4 ounces grapefruit juice, *or* 8 ounces tomato juice, *or* ½ cantaloupe, *or* ½ cup fresh strawberries.

The above list is not intended to be complete. It shows that adequate supplies of the various vitamins can be obtained from ordinary foods.

Meals of good foods are much more pleasant than pills.

Chapter | **16**

# Food, Health, and Disease

The human body has minimal needs for a variety of essential nutrients. We can adapt ourselves to wide ranges of intakes, provided the intake is greater than the minimal need. If the intake of an essential food constituent is below its minimal need, damage will presently result. All the nutrients serve functions in the body. These functions cannot be carried on normally unless the minimal need, at least, is satisfied. Deficiencies will impair health and can lead to definite diseases. In children, growth can be impaired. Obviously, our food intake is one of a number of factors which influence health. The state of the digestive tract is involved since foods must be digested and the products of digestion must be absorbed before these substances can be available for bodily functions. The food we eat is important to attain and maintain health.

A definite lack of food to provide energy lessens the

desire to do work or exercise. We can adapt ourselves to a reduction in calorie intake but part of the adaptation is a lowered energy expenditure in exercise or in work. In concentration camps and in camps for prisoners in the Second World War it was shown that people could adapt themselves and get along remarkably well on food intakes which were much less than customary. One aspect of the survival process was decreased activity.

People can sharply decrease their food intake to lose weight, and this is the only effective method of weight reduction. They will, however, not feel as energetic if the calorie intake is reduced below energy expenditure. A great deal is said in popular articles about the relation of food to vigor, or to tiredness. Factors other than food are involved. Mental attitudes have a great deal to do with vigor. If we want to exercise, or work, we can. If we don't want to do something, we can feel "tired." The amount of rest is important, also. We cannot maintain health and vigor without adequate rest and relaxation. Food intake can be involved in tiredness and in lessened vigor but it is by no means the only influence.

We have a minimal need for protein and the amount needed depends on the kind of protein. If most, or all, of the protein intake is supplied by cereals and vegetables, the amount of protein required is greater than if most of the protein comes from animal-source foods such as milk, cheese, meat, fish, poultry, and eggs. If the minimal need for protein is not met, the maintenance of body protein will be impaired, the protein in the blood will be less than is necessary for health, and presently a diseased state will develop. This is often shown by an accumulation of fluid, or edema. Causes other than pro-

tein deficiency may also bring about an accumulation
of fluid. In most of Africa and in some other areas, lack
of protein is a very serious problem. A disease, kwashiorkor, is produced by protein deficiency. Countries in
which this disease occurs have supplies of food limited
in amount and in variety. If milk were available on the
same generous scale as it is in the "have" countries,
kwashiorkor would not occur—provided people used
milk. In the United States, in Canada, and in Britain
protein deficiency is rare and need not occur because
plenty of good sources of protein are available. We have
noted earlier that the average, per person, daily consumption of protein in these countries is about double
actual need. If you eat the kind of meals recommended
in Chapter 10, you will not need to worry about protein
and you will not need a special kind of breakfast cereal.

A sustained lack of iron will cause one type of anemia.
This type is said to occur more frequently among women
than men, and particularly in women of lower economic
groups. There are other kinds of anemia and in most
of them the adequacy of iron intake is not involved. A
widespread notion is that it is necessary, particularly for
women, to use a pharmaceutical preparation to supply
iron. If generous amounts of meat, eggs, vegetables, and
whole-grain breakfast cereal are eaten the supply of iron
will be at least adequate. The body has a selective arrangement for absorbing iron and it is absorbed accord-
ing to need. When people habitually live on foods having generous amounts of iron, a considerable portion of
the intake may not be absorbed and may be wasted. On
the other hand, a poor selection of food even in "have"
countries can bring about an inadequate supply. Any

difficulty can be prevented by selecting foods sensibly.

In Chapter 3 the diseases which are produced by vitamin deficiencies were described. These diseases have been publicized widely. While pellagra was a serious problem in the Southern states for some years, none of the deficiency diseases are seen frequently in the "have" countries. Unfortunately, many people have received the impression that the only reason for being concerned about food selection is to prevent deficiency diseases. The relation of good food to health is not appreciated.

Good meals are advisable because they are part of the general health picture. Good meals are essential for the healthy growth of children and they constitute one factor for the maintenance of health in adults. Good meals make a difference. You will be less tired in the middle of the morning if you have a decent breakfast. You will be less tired late in the afternoon if you have a decent lunch.

The most prevalent nutrition problem in the highly developed countries is fatness. The cause is the consumption of food having a total calorie value greater than the energy expenditure. Once the habit of overeating has become established it is difficult to break. It is so much easier and wiser not to become a heavy eater. It is possible to enjoy food in moderation. It is possible to enjoy a glass of wine and not become a drunkard and it is equally feasible to be a slim gourmet, and not a fat one. Even if it bores you, I repeat: The best simple advice that can be given is, *a variety of foods in moderation.*

Because habits of food selection and eating begin to develop in early childhood, parents have a responsibility to help children develop good eating habits. There are simple pieces of advice which parents should find useful:

1. A willingness to eat a variety of food and to try new ones will help to prevent feeding problems in childhood, will make life throughout the years more interesting, will help to meet health needs, and for all these reasons should be encouraged.

2. Overeating, even by young children, should be discouraged. Fatness and heaviness, even in babies, is not necessarily a sign of health. There is a widespread tendency to stuff children to make them grow. We don't know what effects rapid growth has in humans but we do know that overfeeding young animals with consequent rapid growth shortens life. Accelerated growth in children has been encouraged in prosperous countries in the last thirty years. It will be twenty to thirty years before information is available as to whether rapid growth was beneficial or harmful. In the meantime, play safe. The habit of overeating, started in childhood and continued in later years leads to fatness—it does shorten life.

3. Examples of good food habits are far more useful than a great deal of talk. If you want your youngster to drink milk, it is wiser for both parents to drink milk—incidentally it will be healthful for everybody. Tommy cannot be expected to use foods which dad refuses or, even worse, ridicules.

It has been noted before in this book that many people have the impression that the choosing of foods to meet health requirements causes meals to be unappetizing. That is, of course, not true and the idea is prevalent because people have not tried good meals. They prefer to keep on following established habits rather than to attempt changes.

It is worth while to consider what changes are needed generally in meals to ensure that health needs are met. One radical change for many people would be to have a good breakfast. I suggest that you try getting up a little earlier and try eating a good breakfast without rushing. The net result will be more beneficial than a few minutes of sleep. That good breakfast may include some foods to which you have not been accustomed. Other changes in your fixed habits may be desirable, also. The drinking of milk may seem so repulsive that you won't even try it. If you do try drinking milk you will presently be glad you did. The use of a wide variety of vegetables may be so unsettling that it just can't be attempted. Well, keep on being a stick-in-the-mud if you are that way. However, meals will be more interesting if there is variety. Even the development of an attitude of trying new foods is rewarding as part of a better attitude to life in general. The Western democracies were not built by sticking to the past.

While it is clear that food intake is a factor in the maintenance of health, and although disease can result from living on meals which fail to meet needs, no promise can be made that a super level of health can be reached by food selection. If your intake of all needed nutrients is now sufficient to meet needs, further increases in intake will not further improve your health.

One other aspect of food selection should be made clear. There are various diseases which are far too prevalent which cannot be related to food use. Many people are greatly worried about cancer. There is no evidence relating any food or any combination of foods to either the production of cancer or to the cure of cancer. If you encounter any claim that certain foods are causes of cancer, don't believe the claims. There is no reason for thinking that a person with cancer can benefit from a special diet. Arthritis is another prevalent and annoying disease. There is no evidence connecting any food or any combination of foods to the development or to the relief of arthritis. If you encounter claims that particular foods help to prevent arthritis, or to cure it, don't believe the claims. There are suspicions that coronary heart disease may be partly caused by using too much fat or by using too much animal fat. At the present time, there is not enough evidence to warrant the advocacy of low-fat meals.

In one sense, food intake is related to the development of several diseases such as diabetes, heart disease and gall-bladder disease. These degenerative diseases have been shown to occur more frequently in fat than in slim people. To help prevent these diseases, it pays to keep slim.

While the wise selection of food will help to maintain health, it cannot be assumed that an unusually high level of health can be produced by nutrition. A claim to this effect is unjustified.

What are the advantages of choosing foods on the basis of meeting bodily needs and of eating healthful meals? These advantages can be stated:

1. Healthful meals, based on good selection, are more economical. Many families could save money.
2. Healthful meals are at least as appetizing and can be more interesting than many customary meals.
3. Healthful meals give healthful growth in children.
4. Healthful meals during pregnancy give healthier babies and help the mother.

5. Healthful meals help to attain and maintain health at any age. Food intake is not the only factor involved in the maintenance of health; it is one factor which we don't need to neglect.

Good food selection means good meals. Good meals are worth eating.

# Index

155

# Date Due